"Clinically applicable, thoroughly researched, and a pleasure to read, this book is a remarkable addition to the child and adolescent literature! For any therapist working with traumatized youth, Shilson brings her respectful, caring approach and pairs it with practical tools. The techniques are useful, easy to follow, creative, and developmentally sensitive. For educators in the field of child therapy, this book brings a thoughtful approach to intervention with the child, their parents, and families, and it grapples with issues that are oftentimes skipped over in child treatment. For seasoned clinicians and students alike, this is a rare find!"

Robert T. Muller, PhD, *author of* Trauma and the Struggle to Open Up *and professor of clinical psychology at York University in Ontario, Canada*

"Kim Shilson has written a brilliant comprehensive text on the therapeutic treatment of traumatized children and adolescents. She includes the basics of diagnosis and assessment, treatment frame, and the therapeutic relationship together with a variety of approaches that represent the best and latest ideas in the field. This is far more than 'just' a book on somatic approaches. It is a necessary addition to the library of every child therapist."

Janina Fisher, PhD, *assistant educational director at Sensorimotor Psychotherapy Institute*

"Kim Shilson has written a valuable resource for any clinician who works with youth. Weaving relevant literature with practical application, she provides a comprehensive overview of how to approach and proceed with youth clients. Her vignettes breathe life into case examples and allow the reader to get a feel for the challenges faced by these young clients. This book is a great guide to a rewarding and meaningful engagement with youth in psychotherapeutic practice, and Kim Shilson illustrates beginning to end the tasks and relationships necessary to work with youth. The presentations of therapeutic options, illustrations, and tables make the work accessible and instantly applicable. An inspiring text."

Rochelle Sharpe Lohrasbe, PhD, *EMDRIA-approved consultant, faculty at Sensorimotor Psychotherapy Institute, and practicing psychotherapist in British Columbia, Canada*

Somatic Methods for Affect Regulation

Somatic Methods for Affect Regulation is a unique resource that presents a variety of approaches for working somatically with youth. Chapters provide an overview of the relevant neuroscience research with a specific focus on affect regulation. The somatic techniques showcased in the book are evidence-based and illustrated with case studies showing their impact. Importantly, the chapters are also full of practical information, including strategies for working with dysregulated youth, information for collaborative and cooperative care, and an appendix with checklists and worksheets to help clinicians plan, guide, and assess their work.

Kimberley L. Shilson, MA, C Psych, is a psychologist in Toronto, Ontario, where she maintains a private practice focusing on assessment and treatment services for traumatized individuals and families. She also provides clinical training and consultation.

Somatic Methods for Affect Regulation

A Clinician's Guide to Healing Traumatized Youth

Kimberley L. Shilson

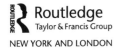
Routledge
Taylor & Francis Group

NEW YORK AND LONDON

First published 2019
by Routledge
52 Vanderbilt Avenue, New York, NY 10017

and by Routledge
2 Park Square, Milton Park, Abingdon, Oxon, OX14 4RN

Routledge is an imprint of the Taylor & Francis Group, an informa business

Library of Congress Cataloging-in-Publication Data
Names: Shilson, Kimberley L., author.
Title: Somatic methods for affect regulation : a clinician's guide
to healing traumatized youth / Kimberley L. Shilson.
Description: New York : Routledge, 2019. |
Includes bibliographical references and index.
Identifiers: LCCN 2018051682 (print) | LCCN 2018052983 (ebook) |
ISBN 9781315213804 (ebook) | ISBN 9781138284425 (hardback) |
ISBN 9781138284432 (pbk.) | ISBN 9781315213804 (ebook)
Subjects: LCSH: Psychic trauma in children–Treatment. |
Child abuse–Treatment. | Child psychology.
Classification: LCC RJ506.P66 (ebook) | LCC RJ506.P66 S55 2019 (print) |
DDC 618.9285/21–dc23
LC record available at https://lccn.loc.gov/2018051682

ISBN: 978-1-138-28442-5 (hbk)
ISBN: 978-1-138-28443-2 (pbk)
ISBN: 978-1-315-21380-4 (ebk)

Typeset in Sabon
by Newgen Publishing UK

Visit the eResources: www.routledge.com/ 9781138284432

This book is dedicated to the memory of my parents, Dolores Ann Jewell and William Henry Shilson.

Contents

PART III
Somatic Interventions: Clinical Applications

PART IV
Special Populations

Figures

Tables

Contributors

Rochelle Sharpe-Lohrasbe, PhD, is an EMDRIA Approved Consultant and provides training internationally as a member of the Sensorimotor Psychotherapy Institute's faculty. Dr. Sharpe also maintains a private practice in Victoria, BC.

Michelle Dick, C. Psych. Assoc., is certified in Somatic Experiencing (SE©). She provides psychological assessment and treatment services at ROCK (Reach Out Centre for Kids) and sees clients in her private practice.

Melanie Cheskes, MSW, RSW, has been working as a clinical social worker for five years, providing counselling services to youth, adults, couples, and families. Melanie also has a Bachelor of Fine Arts and is a talented artist. She was commissioned to do the animal artwork in Figure 12.1.

Acknowledgements

Why am I writing this book now, you ask?

The short answer: In 2016, I was approached to write a book based on a workshop I gave at the ISST-D (International Society for the Study of Trauma and Dissociation) conference in San Francisco. The title of the workshop was "Somatic and Expressive Methods for Healing Traumatized Youth: A Focus on Affect Regulation."

And now the long answer: The ISST-D workshop idea grew out of awareness that my practice was increasingly focused on phase one trauma treatment (safety and stabilization). Given the necessity for some clients to receive short-term trauma treatment, primarily due to lack of financial resources, my practice had somewhat shifted to a focus on phase one trauma treatment and clinical assessment. I was receiving referrals from agencies with limited funding and there were time constraints imposed on the use of funds. These parameters permitted between 9 and 12 sessions. If the traumatic incident was isolated, that is, not complex trauma, some trauma processing could occur within those parameters. However, the assessment process of the majority of clients referred for a particular event, such as a single sexual assault or an incident of internet child exploitation, uncovered multiple areas that were deserving of clinical attention. Fortunately, some of these clients were able to continue treatment following the exhaustion of funding and moved through phases two (trauma processing) and three (integration and reconnection). Over the past few years, I have had the privilege of providing clinical supervision and consultation for service providers at various children's mental health agencies. During the consultations, clinicians frequently requested documentation of the techniques and strategies that I presented. I hope that this book offers creative, somatic strategies for use with dysregulated, traumatized youth and families, and that the strategies can easily be integrated into clinicians' toolboxes.

I had the good fortune to have been introduced to somatic methods about eight years ago at one of Janina Fisher's workshops. Prior to the workshop, I had primarily utilized more structured, less individualized and collaborative approaches (e.g. CBT, TF-CBT, BSFT) in conjunction with play, narrative, and expressive arts interventions. The workshop presented an "a-ha!" moment as I realized this (the body) was the missing piece in trauma work! Subsequently, I went on to train in Sensorimotor Psychotherapy™ (SP), now my primary approach to trauma treatment. I am grateful for the learning and support provided by my mentors at the Sensorimotor Psychotherapy Institute (Ame Cutler, Anne Westcott, and Rochelle Sharpe-Lohrasbe), and SP's founder, Pat Ogden. From SP, I sought additional instruction in body-based frameworks and completed training in SMART, ARC, EMDR, and I attended workshops in the Hakomi and Feldenkrais methods.

Whether you are a seasoned clinician, familiar with the work of brilliant pioneers in the trauma field such as Bruce Perry, Judith Herman, Bessel van der Kolk, and Babette Rothschild, or you are new to working with traumatized youth, my hope is that readers will glean something novel (and interesting!) about the role of affect regulation in trauma work. Further, I hope that you will discover new practical tools and creative interventions to engage, and work with, dysregulated youth and their families.

I greatly appreciate the support of family members and friends who provided me with a quiet space to think and write: Michelle Coombs, Bill Shilson, Marg McKeown, Susan Rosenblum, Ann Haman, Nancy Long, Elsa Monteiro, and Vera Krasovec. To those who gave their precious time and guidance when I initially embarked on this endeavor, thanks to Lynette Danylchuk, Vera Tarman, and Chase Joynt. I am grateful to my colleague and mentor Rochelle Sharpe-Lohrasbe for the words of wisdom and support during this often-grueling writing process. I am thankful to the children and their caregivers who agreed to participate in the production of this project. Note that the youth pictured in the photographs throughout the book are children of friends and colleagues, not clients. It was great fun to hang out and engage with you all in the somatic activities! Last but certainly not least, I am indebted to my friends and colleagues for the care and time spent reviewing drafts of this book – thank you, from the bottom of my heart, Susan Rosenblum, Nancy Long, Tammy Rasmuseen, Elsa Monteiro, Rochelle Sharpe-Lohrasbe, and Vera Krasovec.

Most of all, I owe immense gratitude to the incredibly resilient young people who allowed me to share a portion of their journeys over the past 25 years. You have all touched me profoundly and taught me so much.

Introduction

What is affect regulation and why does it concern those of us who work with traumatized children and adolescents? How is the capacity to regulate affect developed, and how can this development get derailed or stuck? How does the inability to recognize, tolerate, and manage strong emotions or physical sensations impact the developing child? How might dysregulation manifest behaviorally, socially, emotionally, and cognitively? Finally, what can we do to help these youth get back on track?

A lot of questions with few answers at this time. Clinical research is beginning to examine the importance of affect regulation; see, for example, Cloitre et al. (2009) and Ford et al. (2013), and there are both evidence-based practices and emerging treatment models and frameworks that directly address this area in trauma work. As outlined in the first chapter of this book, the child's earliest experiences, including in utero, influence the developing brain, neural networks, and the overall organization of mind–body systems. While attachment is not the subject of this book, one cannot avoid referring to attachment theory when writing about affect regulation since the two processes are intertwined. Indeed, the capacity for affect regulation, as described throughout, is developed through consistent, predictable, and attuned attachment. Additionally, while not the focus of this book, expressive arts methods are peppered throughout since youth are naturally drawn to non-talk, unintimidating methods and they pair well with somatic treatment methods.

Over recent years, my clinical work has increasingly focused on the first component of the phase-oriented treatment model (Herman, 1992). Decades ago, Judith Herman stressed the importance of addressing safety and stabilization prior to working through traumatic memories. More recently, Pat Ogden's model, Sensorimotor Psychotherapy™, and the work of clinical programs at Boston's Justice Resource Institute highlight the primacy of increasing client capacity to recognize, tolerate, and manage emotional and physiological processes before moving into traumatic material. Indeed, Bessel van der Kolk cautions us about the danger of retraumatizing clients by moving too quickly and having them relive the traumatic event by simply "talking about" it (van der Kolk, 2014).

Finally, a quick note on this book's purpose. The material between the covers is intended to expand clinicians' awareness of methods beyond traditional talk therapies, and to see the advantages of incorporating these methods into clinical work with traumatized youth and their caregivers. This book is NOT intended to provide instruction on any of the frameworks or models contained herein; however, I strongly encourage training in any or all of the models as they will enrich your clinical repertoire. As a life-long learner, it sometimes seems like the more I learn, the more I want to know (curiosity is a great quality to have in this field!). With that in mind, perhaps this book is for those who are ready to embark on such a life-long journey.

Organization of This Book

Beyond the Introduction, this book consists of four parts that weave together critical components of effective treatment of complexly traumatized youth: technique and theory, scientist and practitioner (Rothschild, 2000). The four parts are Theory and Somatic Approaches, Essential Components in Clinical Work with Complexly Traumatized Youth, Somatic Interventions – Clinical Applications, and Special Populations. As outlined in the first chapter of this book, the child's earliest experiences, beginning in utero, influence the developing brain, neural networks, and the overall organization of the body–mind system. The material presented within these pages is enriched with interviews peppered throughout, featuring professionals on relevant topics: a Feldenkrais practitioner talks about working with the body's freeze response, a psychotherapist utilizes dance and movement in her treatment of trauma survivors, an Indigenous woman shares her perspective about what mattered after she was taken from her home during the "Sixties Scoop," and a singer/songwriter recounts the healing power of music in her journey. The first chapter provides clinicians with a basic understanding of the use-dependent nature of the developing brain, regions that can be affected by neglect or abuse, and the potentially far-reaching consequences of complex trauma on the individual developing organism. Throughout the book, I will use the terms *clinician* and *therapist* interchangeably to refer to individuals who work with traumatized children and their families (e.g. child and youth workers, social workers, psychologists, school counsellors) for the sake of consistency and brevity.

Safety and stabilization techniques are geared toward an individual client's (or family's) presenting concerns, strengths, and interests. In the late 1800s, Pierre Janet, a French neurologist, described a phase-oriented treatment model for traumatic disorders (van der Hart & van der Kolk, 1989). Decades ago, Judith Herman's phase-oriented model stressed the necessity of addressing safety and stabilization prior to working with traumatic memories (Herman, 1992). More recently, Pat Ogden's Sensorimotor Psychotherapy™, and others such as Dan Siegel and Bessel van der Kolk to name just two, have highlighted the role of helping clients develop resources that increase their capacity to recognize, tolerate, and manage emotional and physiological processes. Van der Kolk has spoken and written extensively about the dangers of retraumatizing a client that is inadequately resourced (e.g. van der Kolk, 2014).

Chapter 1 offers theoretical overviews of neurodevelopment, and trauma and affect regulation. The brain regions identified as crucial in the development of affect regulation, attachment, and as vulnerable to early childhood neglect and abuse, are discussed. Research on inherent neuroplasticity has ushered in hope that clients can overcome the impact of childhood trauma. Models and frameworks have been developed with a focus on repairing developmental injury or re-creating missing early experiences, essentially rewiring the brain in a safe, supportive environment with an attuned, predictable other (i.e. the clinician). This chapter also examines areas of the brain that are implicated in affect regulation and provides an overview of relevant theories such as Porges' Polyvagal Theory, Hebbian theory, and neuroplasticity. There has been a lot of media attention on the ACEs (Adverse Childhood Experiences) study, a longitudinal research project that provides evidence about the long-term impact of childhood trauma (Felitti & Anda, 2005). Furthermore, the relationships between neurodevelopment, attachment theory, and affect regulation are explored. Finally, intergenerational transmission of trauma and epigenetics are introduced in the first chapter.

Chapter 2 describes the frameworks and models that offer a somatic approach, or bottom-up methods, for working with traumatized youth and their caregivers. Research demonstrating the efficacy of the models/frameworks is provided. Case studies are presented in this chapter and they will be referred to throughout the book. The chapter ends with overviews and illustrations of non-somatic models blended with other evidence-based models, namely EMDR and TF-CBT.

Part II begins with Chapter 3, Comprehensive Trauma Assessment. A comprehensive assessment enables us to capture information about concerns and strengths early on so that we can tailor our interventions. Psychoeducation about the process is crucial at the assessment phase and continues throughout treatment. Youth and their caregivers may want to understand why I might suggest a particular exercise to explore and practice (e.g. belly breathing, tapping), based on observations and the assessment, so it is important that we provide the rationale in age-appropriate language. Often, "props" or concrete activities are introduced to help the client grasp the concept and experience the potential effectiveness of the intervention. Guidelines for completion of genograms (aka family trees), time lines, and the use of psychometrics are offered in this chapter. There are a number of guiding principles that facilitate effective treatment of traumatized youth, as reviewed in the fourth chapter. These principles are considered at the beginning, during assessment and engagement processes, and throughout the course of treatment. As discussed in Chapter 5, inclusion of significant others in the child's system, such as caregivers, school staff, and child protection workers, is preferable when working with youth.

By the time children reach my office, they have often received a variety of diagnoses. Complexly traumatized youth are misunderstood and they are frequently diagnosed based on surface symptoms or behavioral presentations. Chapter 6 provides an overview of the diagnoses these youth may have received, such as ADHD, ODD, or Bipolar Disorder, and reviews the symptoms of (overlooked) trauma that may lead to these (mis)diagnoses. This chapter includes a summary of the current criteria for a diagnosis of Complex PTSD (C-PTSD) and provides an overview of a proposed diagnosis that more accurately captures the impact of complex trauma and its presentation in youth: Developmental Trauma Disorder (DTD). Co-morbid diagnoses are also discussed.

Part III delves into the heart of this book: what do we do with all of this information to help the youth? Chapters 7 and 8 address regulation. In Chapter 7, the role of therapist as co-regulator, or surrogate frontal cortex, is explicated. As traumatized or neglected children have typically missed the critical experiences of co-regulation that develop the capacity to tolerate distress and self-soothe, this is a key component in the work with these youth. More often than not, the traumatized youth who have come into treatment reside with caregivers who have their own trauma histories. Thus, the caregivers may not be capable of managing their own affect, let alone facilitating the capacity to self-soothe in a distressed infant. These caregivers may have also inadvertently modeled ineffective or unhealthy coping strategies. In some cases, the therapist must first, or simultaneously, work with caregivers to develop this capacity and, through the processes of modeling and widening the caregiver's window of tolerance, assist caregivers to become interactive regulators for their children. Chapter 8 offers specific strategies to address hyperarousal and hypoarousal in youth. This chapter describes indicators that a child might be outside their window of tolerance (Siegel, 1999) and offers ways the therapist can facilitate movement back to optimal functioning. As Porges (2017) notes, "understanding the response, not the traumatic event, is more critical to the successful treatment of trauma" (p. 56). Thus, it is important that clinicians learn to recognize and work with their clients' indicators. Part III contains two additional chapters, each exploring different ways that the individual's sense of self and safety, and social interactions, may be impacted by trauma. Trauma, by nature, is interpersonal and thus affects our ability to relate to others, to feel safe in relation to others, and shapes the movements and patterns as we move through a social world. Strategies to meet one's needs are learned early in childhood; thus, if a child experiences severe trauma or neglect, the capacity to reach out or protect oneself is impacted on many levels (Ogden, 2006).

The final part addresses youth who face additional challenges, thereby necessitating extra factors to consider in the treatment process. LGBTQ+-identified youth often have unique questions regarding their trauma, and interventions must be tailored to meet the needs of this population. Unique factors are explored and case studies offer a glimpse into the treatment of traumatized LGBTQ+ youth in Chapter 11. Dissociation in traumatized youth, the subject of Chapter 12, has, until recently, been under-recognized and under-reported. Faced with overwhelming fear, abuse, and/or severe neglect, powerless children may tune out their frightening experiences. Over time, repeated use of this defense mechanism may automate and develop into dissociative tendencies. Prolonged, habitual dissociation may lead to the development of "parts" of the self to manage distressing emotions (e.g. rage, despair, shame) while the functioning of daily actions systems (e.g. student, sibling, friend) is maintained. In Chapter 12, the model of structural dissociation (van der Hart, Nijenhuis & Steele, 2006) is introduced, and guidelines about working with dissociative youth are offered. As with earlier chapters, case studies illustrate the incorporation of chapter material.

Glossary of Terms

Since there are numerous concepts used repeatedly throughout this book, let's familiarize ourselves with them now. Should you wish to expand your knowledge on a particular area, and as appropriate, specific resources are cited. Note that there are various definitions and descriptions used for some of these terms; thus the following are summaries or compilations of the definitions as used when I approach my work.

Affect

Affect is the external behavioral presentation of one's emotional state, often displayed through facial expressions, energy levels, motivation, prosody, and movements. Given children's limited vocabulary and ability to express themselves verbally, affect can be observed through their behaviors.

Affect Regulation

Affect regulation refers to the ability to tolerate and manage strong emotional and physiological responses. When the capacity to regulate is optimal or healthy, one can be flexible and adaptive to one's experiences and the demands of the environment. This capacity is compromised in early caregiving where needs are unmet, not met consistently, or dismissed/ignored. With the capacity to regulate, one can express needs, set boundaries, and function well emotionally, cognitively, and socially.

Attachment Style

John Bowlby's seminal work on attachment remains a reference in contemporary research and discussions of attachment theory. He proposed that humans possess an innate drive to form connections with others. Bowlby believed that this instinctive drive was necessary to ensure survival. In the 1970s, Mary Ainsworth's breakthrough work in *The Strange Situation* identified three attachment styles: secure, anxious-avoidant, and anxious-ambivalent. A fourth attachment style, disorganized, was added later. In the experiments, the caregiver left the child in the room with a stranger. Attachment styles were assessed based on behaviors including the child's reaction to the caregiver's departure, the response to the caregiver's return, the child's affective displays, and whether the child could be consoled (if distressed) by the reunion with caregiver. Conclusions suggested that caregiver sensitivity (or attuned responsiveness) to the child's needs engendered the child's attachment style.

Further Reading on Attachment and Attachment Styles

Ainsworth, M., Blehar, M., Waters, E. & Wall, S. (1978). *Patterns of Attachment: A Psychological Study of the Strange Situation*. Hillsdale, NJ: Erlbaum.
Bowlby, J. (1969). *Attachment and Loss: Vol. 1. Attachment*. New York: Basic Books.

There are also YouTube videos on attachment styles featuring Mary Ainsworth, Daniel Siegel, and Alan Schore. Jacob Ham, with animations by Thomas Moon, has created some awesome educational animated videos on attachment.

Attunement

Being in sync on emotional and physical levels. Rhythmic attunement between infant and caregiver is critical to the infant's ability to develop the capacity for self-regulation.

Auxiliary Cortex

When the frontal lobes are off-line and the child (or caregiver) is dysregulated, the clinician may serve as an auxiliary or surrogate cortex. Through interactive regulation, the clinician facilitates growth of the underdeveloped mental processes and structures. Often, especially when working with caregivers, the clinician is bringing the client into the window of tolerance while simultaneously modeling methods to self-regulate. See Ogden, Minton & Pain (2006).

Bottom-Up vs. Top-Down Processing

Cognitive behavioral therapy is an example of a top-down approach. Top-down approaches utilize capacities such as mentalization, memory formation and recall, articulation of thoughts and feelings, problem-solving, and determining cause and effect relationships. These capacities are either undeveloped due to age or developmental level of a child, or they are underdeveloped due to neglect or trauma. With bottom-up approaches, the body is the access point to exploration, processing, and integration of experience. Through increased body awareness, thoughts, feelings, sensations, and core beliefs are accessed.

Further Reading

Ogden, P. & Minton, K. (2000). Sensorimotor Psychotherapy: One Method for Processing Traumatic Memory. *Traumatology*. 6 (3), 149–173.
Ogden, P., Minton, K. & Pain, C. (2006). *Trauma and the Body: A Sensorimotor Approach to Psychotherapy*. New York: W. W. Norton.

Boundaries

Youth who have experienced loose, rigid, or intrusive boundaries may have difficulty in areas such as differentiation of self and other, trusting others, setting limits for self and others, assertiveness, and regulation of affect. Ogden has identified three purposes of boundaries: containment, screening, and protection. Further, there are two types of boundaries to address in treatment: process and physical.

See Ogden & Fisher (2015), Heitzler (2013), and Spinazzola et al. (2011).

Complex Trauma

Sometimes referred to as cumulative trauma, this term is used to describe trauma that occurs repeatedly over a period of time, involving multiple types of traumatic exposure, and is often of an interpersonal nature. Compared to single-incident traumas, such as auto accidents, complex trauma can cause significant disruption in various domains, including emotional, interpersonal, and cognitive development, and can disrupt the development of the capacity to regulate affect. Complex trauma may also lead to distorted or fragmented sense of self.

See Ford & Courtois (2013).

Developmental Trauma Disorder (DTD)

A diagnosis posited by Bessel van der Kolk to capture the myriad of symptomology exhibited by children and youth who have experienced chronic, multiple traumas.

For further information, see Ford et al. (2013), and an article in the *Journal of Canadian Academy of Child and Adolescent Psychiatry* (www.ncbi.nlm.nih. gov/pmc/articles/PMC4032083/pdf/ccap_23_p0142.pdf).

Dissociation

Dissociation is an automatic process wherein unbearable aspects of the trauma are split off or fragmented (e.g. sensations, feelings, thoughts, images, sounds). The traumatic events may not be accessible to conscious memory. Given an infant's inability to use mobilizing defenses such as fight or flight, dissociation may be used to cope with emotional or physical pain. If used repeatedly, this tendency to tune out or disconnect from the self and the overwhelming stimuli may become habituated and have far-reaching detrimental effects on development and functioning.

For further reading see Waters (2016), Fisher (2017), and Wieland (2015).

DSM-5 (Diagnostic and Statistical Manual of Mental Disorders, *5th Edition*)

A publication of the American Psychiatric Association, this is considered the most comprehensive resource manual for diagnosis and classification of mental health used by clinicians and researchers. The criteria for PTSD changed from the DSM IV-TR to reflect the greater impact fewer symptoms can have on children and youth (Ford & Courtois, 2013, p 131). Van der Kolk and colleagues' efforts, through field trials, to include a diagnosis specific to children and youth (Developmental Trauma Disorder – DTD) did not succeed; however, many clinicians refer to DTD when discussing assessment and treatment of traumatized youth. Perhaps DTD will be included in the next edition of the DSM.

Dual Awareness

This quality is necessary in order to safely work through the trauma. Dual awareness involves being in the present, with the therapist, while attending to the traumatic memory or fragment as it unfolds in the present moment.

Felt Sense

Eugene Gendlin referred to the body's intuitive awareness as "felt sense" in his technique Focusing. Felt sense is the ability to access nonverbal, sensory, or somatic information. Somatic clinicians facilitate clients' awareness of their "felt sense" and trust in the wisdom of the body. The felt sense is the quality of sensations (e.g. fluttery, tight, or heavy), temperatures, or even colors in the body. As Gendlin noted: "Your body 'knows' the who of each of your situations – vastly more aspects of it than you can think" (Gendlin, 1978, p. viii). Through increased body awareness, clients can then choose or change their responses.

Hyperarousal

Hyperarousal refers to excessive activation in the nervous system, specifically the sympathetic branch of the nervous system. This may be present as high physical activity, fleeting thoughts, shaking of the limbs/body, anxious behavior, verbose and tangential speech, and impulsivity.

Hypoarousal

Hypoarousal refers to a very low level of activation, specifically activation of the parasympathetic nervous system. Individuals who are hypoaroused may appear lethargic, sad, lack cognitive and verbal abilities, lack motivation, and may report feeling numb or dead inside.

Implicit Messages

Implicit messages are messages that children internalize about themselves that are not directly expressed by the caregiver. For example, children whose caregivers are distant or emotionally unavailable may come to view themselves as unworthy of love and affection. Present and attuned caregiving experiences convey implicit messages that a child is valued and loved.

Interoception

Awareness that occurs at a physiological level. Porges notes that "interoception reflects the feedback from our viscera to our brain" (Porges, 2017, p. 142). Interoception occurs within consciousness and is an important capacity in decision-making, especially when faced with a potentially unsafe situation. Youth with early or complex trauma histories, having disconnected from or numbed body awareness, may lack the capacity to tune in and respond to their visceral responses.

See Ogden, Minton and Pain (2006) and Porges (2017) for more on interoception.

Interpersonal Neurobiology (IPNB)

Dan Siegel is the trailblazer in this field. IPNB combines various sciences (e.g. biology, psychology, anthropology) to increase our understanding of human development and the human experience, particularly in relation to other humans. Basically, IPNB is the integration of our inner experiences in connection with others on a neurobiological level.

See Mindsight.org and a quick introduction by Siegel on YouTube (https://youtu.be/JeGBhVm13mc).

Mindfulness

There are many definitions for mindfulness. For this book, mindfulness is defined as the capacity to be fully present in the present moment, and able to calmly observe moment-by-moment experience.

For detailed descriptions and definitions, refer to the works by Ogden, Siegel and van der Kolk listed in the References.

Mirror Neurons

Mirror neurons are activated when we have a reaction (physiological, motoric, emotional) that is similar to what we observe in another person. For example, when someone smiles, we tend to smile back. Mirror neurons are important in child development as they reflect attunement and facilitate the capacity to self-regulate. For example, when a baby appears distressed or cries and her caregiver reflects that distress (validates the baby's state), the baby learns that her feelings are valid, and that her caregiver cares for her. As a result, the baby learns to self-regulate and internalizes a positive sense of self.

Both Bruce Perry and Dan Siegel have written extensively about mirror neurons. See also Iacoboni (2008) and Iacoboni & Mazziotta (2007).

Mobilizing Defenses, Immobilizing Defenses

Humans are wired to defend themselves from risk. Mobilizing defenses are fight and flight, and immobilizing defenses are freeze and the feigned death response. Babies cannot defend themselves with mobilizing actions and thus may react to threat with a freeze response. The freeze response is a state of high activation of the sympathetic nervous system paired with immobility. Similarly, young children may not be able to fight or flee a threatening situation or person and may cope with overwhelming situations by freezing or collapsing/aka feigned death response.

Refer to the work of Pat Ogden and Peter Levine for more information.

Neuroception

Neuroception occurs below conscious awareness. Unlike interoception, we are unaware of what is causing our nervous systems to activate or calm. With youth, I often refer to this process as the spidey senses tingling when they sense that something is not right or there is risk.

Neuroplasticity

Neuroplasticity, defined by Siegel (2007) as the mind's capacity to be altered by experience, offers opportunity for growth through therapeutic interaction and activity. Similarly, Doidge (2007) posits, in his seminal book *The Brain That Changes Itself*, that the brain is not a hard-wired machine as once believed, and that the brain's structure and function can be shaped or molded over the course of our lifetimes. Thus, regardless of the pruning (apoptosis) of under- or undeveloped brain structures or regions due to earlier experiences of neglect or abuse, the potential for growth exists.

Procedural Learning

After repetition, actions are learned and automated. For example, most adults are able to tie their shoelaces without conscious awareness. Through practice, learning is accomplished via activation and integration of motor and cognitive processes.

Proprioception

Awareness of the position of one's body through muscles and joints, and proprioception informs us about our position in space. Proprioceptive input might include pressure or weight. Some clients, for example, like to place a weighted blanket or cushion on their laps when they arrive because they find this calming.

Prosody

Prosody refers to the rhythm, intonation, and tone of the voice. The therapist can use their prosody to co-regulate and enhance neuroception of safety.

Proximity

Proximity refers to nearness or distance in terms of space. Somatic therapists may engage clients in mindful experiments to explore their boundaries vis-à-vis proximity.

PTSD (Post-traumatic Stress Disorder)

The DSM-5 added criteria beyond the symptoms reexperiencing, avoidance, and hyperarousal seen in previous versions. Essentially, a distorted view of self and the world has been added. Briefly, the criteria for PTSD in the DSM-5 are:

A. Exposure to death (actual or threatened), severe injury, or sexual violence.
B. Presence of intrusive symptoms such as nightmares, flashbacks, or physiological reactions (source may be unknown to the survivor). Note: In children, there may be repetitive play, nightmares with indiscernible content, or play that contains reenactments of the trauma.
C. Avoidance of reminders of the event(s), such as locations, people, thoughts.
D. A negative shift in mood and cognitions following the event(s).
E. Significant changes in reactivity or arousal (e.g. hypervigilance, feeling "on edge," sleep difficulties) after the traumatic event(s).

Please refer to the DSM-5 for a full description of criteria and their indicators.

Somatic

Somatic means body-related. Somatic psychotherapies are bottom-up therapies, which means they use the body as an entry point to explore sensations and related thoughts and feelings.

Trauma

An individual is traumatized when their system is overwhelmed by an experience, often with the threat of death of self or an attachment figure. Van der Kolk and Fisler (1995) described traumatization as an experience of an inescapable stressful event that overwhelms one's existing coping mechanisms. Note that the subjective experience of the event matters, as one person might be traumatized by a bike accident, for example, while another person might get up, dust himself off, and carry on with his ride. Also note that not everyone who experiences a traumatic event develops PTSD (post-traumatic stress disorder). In terms of presentation and diagnosis, trauma can been divided into subtypes:

•   acute trauma

An acute trauma is usually a single episode or incident. Examples include serious auto accidents, and witnessing a violent attack on your way home. While there may be intense fear, feelings of overwhelm, a sense of helplessness, nightmares or flashbacks, symptoms typically subside within three months.

- chronic trauma

Chronic trauma is repeated trauma, such as ongoing physical or sexual abuse.

- complex trauma

Judith Herman (1992) first proposed Complex PTSD as distinct from PTSD. Courtois (2004) noted: "Complex trauma generates complex reactions, in addition to those currently included in the DSM-IV." In addition to avoidance, reexperiencing (e.g. nightmares and flashbacks), and hypervigilance seen in a diagnosis of PTSD, complex trauma includes disturbances in the following areas:

1. Regulation – difficulty managing emotions such as anger and sadness, possible suicidal thoughts with persistent sadness.
2. Consciousness – forgetting or reliving the traumatic event(s), possibly occurrences of feeling detached from the body or cognitive processes (dissociation).
3. Distorted self-perception and world view – feelings of helplessness and shame or guilt, and loss of faith leading to hopelessness.
4. Interpersonal relationships – difficulties with trust and being in relationship with others.

Trauma-Focused Treatment

Trauma-focused treatment recognizes and highlights the impact of the child's trauma on emotional cognitive, behavioral, and physical development and safety. This approach strives to provide education to child and caregiver about the impact of trauma, and offers skills to assist the child (and caregiver) to cope with feelings, sensations, and cognitions associated to the traumatic experience.

According to SAMHSA (Substance Abuse and Mental Health Services Administration, www.samhsa.gov), trauma-specific interventions recognize:

1. the survivor's need to be respected, informed, connected, and hopeful regarding their own recovery;
2. the interrelation between trauma and symptoms of trauma such as substance abuse, eating disorders, depression and anxiety;
3. the need to work in a collaborative way with survivors, family and friends of the survivor, and other human service agencies in a manner that will empower survivors and consumers.

Trauma-Informed Care

There is a movement toward trauma-informed care with the recognition among helping professionals that cumulative and complex trauma frequently underlie many presenting concerns and mental health issues.

> According to SAMHSA (www.samhsa.gov), a trauma-informed approach encompasses the following:
>
> 1. recognizes the signs and symptoms of trauma in clients, families, staff, and others involved with the system;
> 2. responds by fully integrating knowledge about trauma into policies, prcedures, and practices; and
> 3. seeks to actively resist retraumatization.

The BC Provincial Mental Health and Substance Use Planning Council stress the importance of distinguishing trauma-informed services from trauma-specific treatment. Their Trauma Informed Practice (TIP) Guide (2013) notes that trauma-informed services work at "the client, agency and staff levels from the core principles of: trauma awareness, safety; trustworthiness, choice and collaboration; and building strengths and skills," whereas trauma-specific services "are offered in a trauma-informed environment and are focused on treating trauma through therapeutic interventions involving practitioners with specialist skills" (p. 4).

Truncated

A truncated action is one that has not been completed. In Sensorimotor Psychotherapy™, for example, we may work with preparatory movements suggestive of an action that wanted to happen. Ogden (2009) notes: "In a sensorimotor approach, clients are helped to rediscover their truncated physical defensive impulses to push away, strike out, or run—actions that were not executed during the abuse." (p. 8).

For example, if a child was physically abused growing up and froze during the assaults due to the inability to fight back or flee, there may be movements such as pushing away or running away that were truncated.

Vestibular

The vestibular system is connected to the inner ear, and this system detects balance. With somatic methods, we can work with a child's vestibular system to improve poor balance that may be impacting functioning, such as playing games with peers or even simply walking across a room. Children who seek vestibular input like to swing, sit/bounce on physio balls, spin in chairs, or bounce on trampolines.

Window of Tolerance (WOT)

This concept was introduced by Dan Siegel (1999) to describe the fluctuations in arousal (hyper, hypo) often experienced by trauma survivors. There is an optimal zone within which the individual has the capacity to think, feel, sense, and act in coordinated, coherent ways. Above or below this window, one is unable to absorb or integrate stimuli and thus cannot take in therapeutic material. The WOT is different for each client and must be explored and understood at the beginning of treatment if treatment is to be useful. The WOT has been referred to as "bandwidth," and other experts use different terms for the same concept: "Modulation Model" (Ogden), "Window of Receptivity" (Wieland).

Complex Trauma Vignettes

Note: All of the youth in these complex trauma case studies are composites of multiple clients. In order to protect the confidentiality of clients and families, identifying information has been changed or fictionalized.

Adele

Adele, 13, was referred for services by a local victim services agency. She had been the victim of sexual exploitation on the internet. Adele initially presented as a petite, self-assured, outgoing girl. She did not understand why people were concerned about what transpired during the internet interactions with an adult male. Ongoing investigations revealed that there were four similar incidents with men on the internet that she had not disclosed to anyone.

Adopted from war-torn Kosovo at 14 months of age, it was love at first sight for her adoptive, middle-class parents. Initial meetings and assessment suggested that Adele likely suffered the effects of Alcohol-Related Neurodevelopmental Disorder (ARND). Little was known about Adele's biological parents except that she had been removed from the care of them due to their inability to care for her. Adele presented with a range of challenges including learning difficulties, adaptive and social skill deficits, sensory issues, poor decision-making skills vis-à-vis cause and effect, and she struggled with affect regulation. Adele attended a school for students with learning disabilities. At school, she was considered high functioning, was well liked by school personnel, and she was often given leadership roles. She reveled in having the control and responsibility the leadership roles entailed. When it got to be too much, however, Adele could not say no as she did not do well with conflict and she did not know how to set boundaries. She tended to isolate herself from her peers, other than a couple of friends in one class. The friendships were sporadic on and off due to Adele's inability to manage conflict and her successive retreats from interpersonal interaction.

Adele's distorted self-concept and low self-esteem made her vulnerable to the bullying and online victimization that she experienced. Her impulsivity and poor regulation skills contributed to self-injurious behavior (cutting and burning), suicidal thoughts (no plan or attempts), and romantic involvement with girls that were more severely dysregulated than her. Adele shared that she self-identified as bisexual and reported that she was equally interested in boys and girls. Woven throughout treatment was psychoeducation about sexual abuse, healthy relationships (peer, romantic, and family), and neurodevelopment, attachment and trauma. The many challenges of working with this girl's complex trauma will be expanded upon in Chapters 5 and 7.

Vincent

Vincent was 14 years old when he was referred for counseling through a victim services program for youth. He got involved with the agency following disclosure that he had been sexually assaulted by an adult male that he had met through an online hookup site. Prior to our first meeting, Vincent had received counseling services and been hospitalized twice. His parents, an intact heterosexual couple of Portuguese descent, were supportive loving parents. They worked hard to navigate the disconnected, often homophobic, systems to get support for their son.

When I met Vincent, he was no longer suicidal, but he was experiencing symptoms of anxiety and depression, and he was regularly using substances (weed and alcohol). He was experiencing eating challenges due to body image issues, and his sleep was severely disrupted. Though Vincent was easily engaged, he was guarded and his body was often taut, contorted like a pretzel as he sat across the room in his chair. Sometimes his leg shook rapidly throughout the sessions and his eye contact was limited. When discussing emotionally charged material, Vincent's eyes grew wide and he had a tick-like action with his mouth. Vincent's range of affect was also limited, his face blank or, alternately, apprehensive.

Prior to the sexual assault, Vincent had been doing well academically and he had positive interactions with his family most of the time. His relationship with his sister, two years younger, was typical, with occasional bouts of sibling rivalry interspersed with supportive connection. He had a lot of friends, was physically active, and enjoyed life. Drastic changes in Vincent's behavior, mood, and relationships followed the assault. Despite having a relatively secure base, Vincent's experience is one of complex trauma. His healing journey will be discussed in Chapters 2, 5, 6, 7, 8, and 11.

Lake

Lake and their family were referred by a colleague to address dissociation and gender-identity issues. Upon meeting, Lake informed me that they had Dissociative Identity Disorder and they were transgender. Lake stated a preference for they or him/he pronouns. Lake was 15 years old and the second child of an intact, mixed-race heterosexual couple. They did not get along with their older brother. Initial meetings and assessment revealed that Lake had not experienced any historical childhood trauma.

Academically, Lake was an average student. Peer relationships were often strained and Lake had difficulty maintaining friendships. Lake often presented as immature and impulsive and was prone to emotional outbursts. Lake vacillated between clingy, needy behaviors to complete shut-down and disconnection. There was a history of engaging in self-injurious behaviors and suicidal talk. Lake was easily engaged and possessed a variety of interests and skills that facilitated the treatment process. Furthermore, Lake was well-versed on their symptoms and challenges as they had done their own research via the internet. Over time, we learned that there was an incident that occurred at a very young age. Lake's trauma history and the challenges of working with this young person will be discussed in Chapter 12.

Dee

Dee, 14, was referred by a colleague for assessment and treatment due to concerns related to mood, school refusal, "oppositional behavior," self-injury, and substance use. Dee came from a home where she was exposed to domestic violence and caregiver substance use from an early age. She also had a much older brother that terrorized and physically and verbally abused her. Dee never knew her father. Her mother was a hard-working single parent with a proclivity to engage in unhealthy relationships with men. During the assessment, Dee shared that she skipped school because she was too anxious, and that she had recently gotten interested in smoking weed. Although Dee was charming, witty, and likeable, teachers were exasperated with her mood swings and truancy. When Dee began treatment, she self-identified as queer and nonbinary, and over the course of treatment she would experiment with how she physically presented herself as well as partnering with boys and girls.

During the assessment process, Dee disclosed that she had been sexually abused by an elderly uncle from the ages of 5 through 8. She shared that although she had told family members at the time, she was not believed and the abuse was never reported. Additionally, she had seen two practitioners before me and there was no exploration or reporting of the alleged abuse. I surmised that the lack of validation, and the abuse itself, contributed to Dee's "presenting concerns." Following the disclosure, I reported the alleged abuse to child protection services and we spent some time in treatment, sometimes conjointly with mother, addressing the impact of the abuse and lack of validation.

Dee had a lot of anger, sadness, and confusion in relation to her family and her past. She was quite intelligent but severely dysregulated. Her dysregulation impacted her abilities, her self-concept, and her motivation. She traveled a fair distance independently to attend sessions and she was consistent with attendance. She also had many skills and qualities that surfaced over the course of treatment and were used to strengthen her sense of self, and her motivation to move through her traumatic experiences. Dee's healing journey will be shared in Chapters 5, 6, 7, 10, and 12.

Dylan

Dylan was 7 years old when he was referred to a children's mental health agency by child protection services (CPS). He was a mixed-race boy living with his mother and grandmother. Dylan came to the attention of CPS due to problematic behaviors at school: he would not remain seated in the classroom, he refused to use the public restrooms, he was highly active and inattentive, and he was aggressive toward peers and his teacher. When CPS interviewed Dylan's mother, a single parent, they learned that he was aggressive with her as well and she struggled with managing his behavior at home.

During the assessment process, Dylan shared an incident of sexual abuse by an older male cousin. The incident was not seen as sexual abuse and had not been reported. The incident was considered rough play between family members. I made a report and CPS followed up with the family. Dylan and his caregivers required a lot of psychoeducation and parenting skills. His mother participated in sessions to learn coping skills so that she could regulate herself as well as her son. Dylan was easily engaged, playful, and athletic. He came into the agency's program as part of a city-wide research project on the effectiveness of TF-CBT. Working within the model's protocol was at times challenging with this youngster. I was forced to be creative and involve more movement than was typically used with the model, so somatic and play methods were blended into treatment with Dylan and his caregivers. The blended approach taken to address Dylan's complex trauma will be detailed in Chapter 2.

Kevin

By the age of 10, Kevin had received multiple diagnoses and participated in many treatment programs. He was living with his mother in the midst of a contentious divorce. His mother openly expressed her hatred for Kevin's father, and she frequently reminded Kevin how similar he was to his father. Kevin had a younger sister who he was protective toward, but he was frequently admonished for aggression toward peers at school. He was also identified as "gifted" at school. His mother complained that he did not like affection and refused hugs. Kevin had no friends at school or in the community.

Kevin was not easy to engage. He made no eye contact, muttered when he spoke (if he spoke), and clearly did not wish to be in treatment. Kevin was quite small for his age. I noticed his slumped posture, sunken chest, frequent sighs, and heavy gait immediately, and I knew that his body was telling a story that he could not express with words. Part of Kevin's journey will appear in Chapters 9 and 10.

Mateo

Mateo was an 11-year-old boy referred to an agency by child protection services involved with his adoptive family. Mateo had been in an orphanage for the first 5 years of his life. After the referral, the family received counseling services. Due to his adoptive mother's limited English, I worked closely with a clinician from another agency to provide services in their language. Following observation of Mateo in his school setting, it was agreed that he was not doing well in the large classroom, and we enrolled him in the agency's school-based program. Mateo was initially involved with the TF-CBT city-wide project; however, it became apparent quickly that Mateo and his family would need more intensive treatment.

Mateo presented with flat affect and he frequently tuned out during conversation and in the classroom. He was prone to aggressive verbal and physical outbursts. When classroom staff confronted him about his behavior, he denied having engaged in the activity. Staff grew increasingly frustrated with Mateo and he was frequently restrained or isolated from the group. Psychoeducation about trauma was offered to school staff to encourage them to respond to him differently. Eventually, Mateo was removed from the school program, and he was put in residential care because his adoptive parents could no longer tolerate his lying, hoarding of food, and other concerning behaviors. The challenges of working with this youngster's trauma history and the many systems involved in his care are chronicled in Chapters 4 and 5.

Part I

Theory and Somatic Approaches

1 Brain Development, Trauma, and Affect Regulation

> An understanding of the neurobiology of trauma may further enhance our conceptualization of the long-term sequelae of trauma and help guide our therapeutic efforts toward increasing the accuracy and specificity of clinical interventions.
>
> (Pat Ogden, 2006, p. 139)

Research in the field of neurobiology has shown that the capacity for self-regulation depends on early experiences with an attuned caregiver. Moreover, recent research has identified specific brain regions and mechanisms impacted by child abuse and neglect. Before a child is born, the brain and body are creating crucial connections. Through processes of use-dependent growth and pruning of dendrites and neuronal networks, the early brain takes shape. Siegel has expanded the use-dependent notion to "use-expectant" (Siegel, 2007). At birth, the infant already has over 85 billion neurons, and the first couple of years are critical to optimal development.

Clinical experts and researchers in neurobiology have written about the bottom-up development of critical areas and functions of the brain. That is, the more primitive parts of the brain responsible for unconscious processes, such as respiration, breathing, and heart rate, are the first to develop. As reflected in the opening quote, the work of Pat Ogden and other somatic healers recognizes that trauma work must consider neurobiology, and that interventions tailored to the individual from a bottom-up approach may have the greatest impact. Bruce Perry's diagram (see Figure 1.1) offers a visual representation of neurodevelopment and the key functions of these areas. Structured akin to an upside down pyramid, with greater mass and complexity on the upper layers (cortex), basic functions are on the bottom and, as the brain grows based on maturation and life experience, the capacities for more intricate processes (e.g. problem-solving, decision-making) are at the top. This is simplistic as there is interconnection between the areas; however, the important fact is that the development of higher functions depends on the development of the lower level areas.

Even more simplistic is Canadian neuroscientist Paul MacLean's triune brain model (see Figure 1.2 below). According to the triune brain model, the human brain is composed of three interconnected areas that MacLean referred

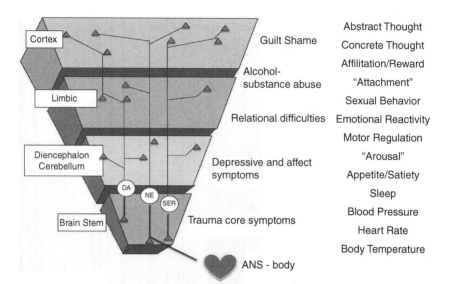

Figure 1.1 Bottom-up Brain Development
Source: Bruce D. Perry (2017). Image used with permission.

to as the reptilian brain (brain stem and cerebellum), the limbic system (also referred to as the emotional brain), and the neocortex (also referred to as the thinking brain). These areas develop in a bottom-up, use-dependent manner. From the brain stem up, patterns are formed and capacities are developed. If development is impeded at a lower area, upper areas can be profoundly impacted. Regions within the limbic system, such as the amygdala and hippocampus that are involved in functions such as memory and emotions, may not develop optimally if there is trauma or insufficient experience to facilitate growth of the lower regions. Another important concept in brain development is the well-known expression *what fires together wires together*. This concept, known as Hebbian theory, was introduced in Donald Hebb's 1949 book *The Organization of Behavior: A Neuropsychological Theory*. Hebb's theory provided an explanation about learning as a product of neuronal firing patterns and continues to be referenced in the works of current neuropsychological theorists (Cozolino, 2006; Heller & LaPierre, 2012; Siegel, 2003).

From a trauma perspective, if the child experiences neglect that impedes the development of his capacity to self-soothe, he may encounter difficulties in areas such as learning, social interaction, and mood disturbances. If the neglect continues over years, the resultant complex trauma might manifest in the use of substances or self-injurious behaviors as attempts to regulate, difficulties in the ability to form close, trusting relationships, or early dropout from school due to inability to focus and retain material. The ACEs study, discussed later in this chapter, illuminates the long-term, far-reaching vicissitudes of childhood trauma.

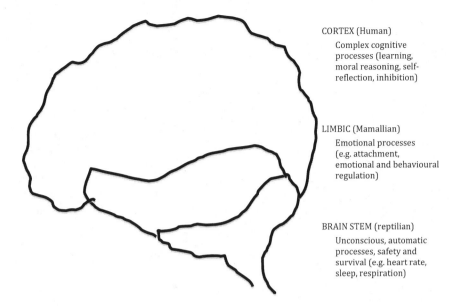

CORTEX (Human)
Complex cognitive
processes (learning,
moral reasoning, self-
reflection, inhibition)

LIMBIC (Mamallian)
Emotional processes
(e.g. attachment,
emotional and behavioural
regulation)

BRAIN STEM (reptilian)
Unconscious, automatic
processes, safety and
survival (e.g. heart rate,
sleep, respiration)

Figure 1.2 The Triune Brain

What promotes optimal development of these early connections? Much has been written on the role of attunement in early brain development (Ford et al., 2013; Perry, 2009; Sroufe, 1995; Stein & Kendall, 2003). Attunement during the child's first relationship, with the primary attachment figure, is crucial to brain development. Through mimicking or mirroring the baby's state, whether the baby is distressed or happy, and accurately responding to the baby, and recognizing whether the baby's cry is a call for connection, hunger, to soothe, or to change a diaper, the caregiver calms the baby's nervous system and instills a sense of safety. As the caregiver regulates the infant, she learns that it is acceptable to have needs and that she can reach out (i.e. proximity seeking) to have those needs met. She also learns that she is worthy of the love and affection that she receives from her caregiver. Of course, there will be times when the caregiver is misattuned or unable to meet the infant's need immediately, but through sequences of rupture and repair the infant develops tolerance and trust that her needs will be met. This is moving into attachment theory so we will move on to other factors that promote crucial neurobiological development.

Gaskell and Perry state:

The crucial regulatory neural networks involved in the stress response (and multiple other functions) are themselves modulated through patterned, repetitive, and rhythmic input from both bottom-up (i.e., somatosensory) and top-down (i.e., cerebromodulatory) systems.

(in Malchiodi & Crenshaw, 2014, p. 184)

Rhythm is built into the brain stem and occurs below conscious awareness. We are not aware of our heart beating or breathing, for example, but these rhythms are crucial to our survival and facilitate functions in higher brain regions. One need only look at an infant attempting to self-soothe though rocking side to side to witness the fundamental role rhythm plays in our lives. Rhythm is used in interactive regulation as well, when the caregiver rocks the baby or walks around making cooing sounds, for example. In addition to the rhythmic input, the caregiver's prosody plays a role in brain development, specifically the instillation of capacity for self-regulation. The caregiver's soothing tone and pace settles the nervous system and creates a sense of safety and well-being in the infant (Ogden, 2006). Prosody, along with movement and facial expressions, are components of implicit communication essential to optimal neurological, social, and emotional growth. Janina Fisher has described this process as interactive neurobiological regulation (Fisher, 2010).

ACEs (Adverse Childhood Experiences) Study

In 1998, Vincent Felitti and colleagues published a ground-breaking longitudinal study on the long-term, far-reaching impact of child abuse (Felitti et al., 1998). Felitti had been conducting research in an obesity clinic when he became curious about the high dropout rate of patients who successfully lost weight in the program. Upon exploration, he uncovered histories of sexual abuse that had not been addressed in treatment, primarily because the right questions were not asked. This longitudinal study, a joint project between Kaiser Permanente and the CDC, initially conducted between 1995 and 1997 with over 17,000 participants, provided evidence for a direct link between childhood maltreatment and various adult social, emotional, cognitive, and psychological problems. Adult health issues ranged from mental illness, to addictions, to medical issues such as heart disease and early mortality. The ACEs study is significant given the large sample size, the longitudinal nature of the research, and the demonstrated links between early child abuse and a vast range of adult health issues, and the results have been cited by many contemporary trauma experts.

Most alarming, the research demonstrated a cumulative effect of multiple exposures to trauma. Adverse life experiences included in the survey were items such as emotional, physical, or sexual abuse, and living in a household with mentally ill caregivers or domestic violence. Here is a sample of the staggering statistics:

- Life expectancy was reduced by 20 years, from 80 to 60, for those with six or more ACEs.
- Those with four or more ACEs were 2.2 times more likely to have heart disease than those with none.
- Individuals with four or more ACEs were 12.2 times more likely to have ever attempted suicide than responders with none.

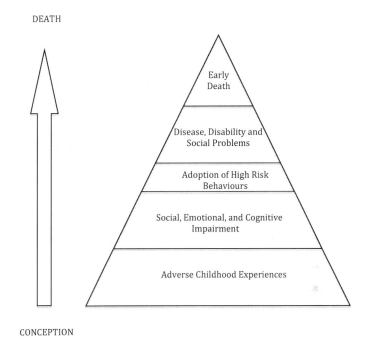

Figure 1.3 ACE Pyramid
Source: Adapted from www.cdc.gov/violenceprevention/acestudy/ACE_graphics.html.

As with most research, there are limitations to the study that are beyond the scope of this book. There is a website with an abundance of material on the study for those who wish to learn more about ACEs (www.acestoohigh.com). The ACEs study is included here because it highlights how medical professionals often overlook historical factors that may contribute to presenting symptoms reflecting dysregulation, how widespread childhood trauma is in our society, and the vast ramifications of unrecognized, untreated childhood trauma. Findings suggest a paradigm shift in how clinicians conduct assessments: ask "what happened to you?" rather than "what's wrong with you?"

Neuroplasticity – Hope for Healing!

As noted above, neurons that fire together, wire together. With this concept in mind, we know that with repetition and rhythm (Perry, in Malchiodi & Crenshaw, 2014) new connections can be formed and strengthened. Siegel (2007) wrote: "Neuroplasticity is the term used when connections change in response to experience." (p. 30). Thus, there is a possibility for children who have experienced severe neglect, for example, to generate or regenerate neuronal growth in under- or undeveloped brain regions. The concept of neuroplasticity is important in work with traumatized youth and families because it gives us hope and, more significantly, offers hope to the youth and caregivers that feel hopeless about the possibility for healing.

The Burgeoning Field of Interpersonal Neurobiology (IPNB)

Moving from the Brain to the Mind

Siegel describes the field of interpersonal biology as a combination of fields, such as anthropology, education, psychology, and neurology, "into one view of the nature of being human" (Siegel & Solomon, 2013, p. 1), a view that includes the mind, relationships, human development, and general wellness. "The capacity of caregivers to modulate physiologic arousal reinforces the child's attachment to them and allows a smooth alternation between activities that increase and reduce arousal as they go back and forth between exploring the environment and returning to their mothers" (van der Kolk, 2003, p. 295). Perry (2002) has outlined six core strengths that are sequentially developed through effective clinical work with traumatized youth:

1. attachment – the ability to form a dyadic relationship with another, typically a primary caregiver;
2. self-regulation – the ability to self-regulate depends on the earlier attachment relationship;
3. affiliation – learn how to be connected with other people, cannot be mastered without ability to self-regulate;
4. attunement – noticing others are different from oneself and learning what others are like;
5. tolerance – through learning and attunement, appreciating individual difference;
6. respect – beyond tolerating differences, recognition that the world needs diversity and we are stronger with diversity.

Based on these core strengths, the attachment relationship precipitates the capacity for self-regulation that is necessary for us to function in our social world. The youth we see in our practices have either gotten stuck or have underdeveloped attachment and self-regulation. This book focuses on ways to rewire or build these capacities through enhancing regulation.

Social interest and awareness about the role of the brain in mental health and interconnectedness was evident in the Brain Project. The project's goals were to promote and support a local brain health and aging program. I was particularly intrigued by Charmaine Lurch's piece, entitled *Cognectica* (see Figure 1.4), one of 100 sculptures on display throughout the city in 2017. The accompanying blurb read: "This sculpture, Cognectica, addresses connectivity – how we build and expand our brains through encounters with each other. These connections – both physical and emotional – create a topography that

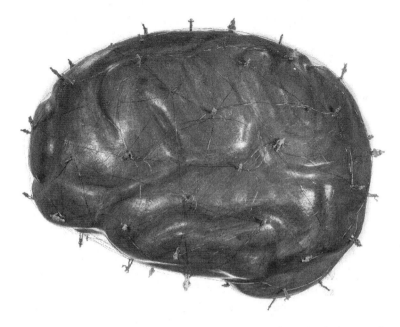

Figure 1.4 Contemporary Artwork Reflecting the Significance of the Mind–Body–Social Connection

Source: "Cognectica" by Charmaine Lurch.

maps our way of being in the world." Wow, I just had to meet this woman and learn more about her work and her process. The interdisciplinary artist, arts researcher, and educator agreed to meet me and subsequently granted permission to include her work in this book. For me, her piece speaks to the importance of connection, highlighted in the writings of experts in the field such as Perry and Siegel, and the reciprocal impact of our minds and relationships: our minds shape and are shaped by connection.

Key Brain Regions and Structures

Amygdala

This is a small, almond-shaped mass within the limbic system. The amygdala is involved in emotional processing, particularly in relation to survival, and memory storage. It has been referred to as the alarm system of the brain because it receives sensory input via the brain stem. Badenoch (2008) notes that the amygdala "tells us when to pay attention and makes a preliminary evaluation" (p. 16) about whether incoming information is safe or not.

LeDoux (1996) writes about the high road and the low road. It takes only 12 milliseconds for the thalamus to process sensory input and signal the alarm system (the amygdala); however, it takes 30–40 milliseconds to reach the prefrontal cortex where thinking and analysis of the input occurs. He calls the former the low road (emotional brain), and the latter the high road (thinking brain). In traumatizing experiences, and when being triggered or caught in a flashback of the trauma, there is no access to the prefrontal cortex (PFC). The brain responds quickly to stimuli, often through neuroception of danger whether it is past or present, and the capacity to think is lost. Siegel's "Flip Your Lid" and hand model of the brain provide an accessible way for children and youth, and their caregivers, to understand what is happening when the child seems to be "misbehaving" when they are in fact dysregulated and their frontal lobes are off-line. See Siegel's hand model of the brain on YouTube – https://youtu.be/gm9CIJ74Oxw.

Prefrontal Cortex (PFC)

The PFC is the last part of the brain to mature. Functions of the PFC include impulse control, complex and moral reasoning, and working memory. Somatic psychotherapies recognize that mindfulness engages the PFC and this is how changes in patterned responses take shape. When a person is being traumatized or experiencing flashbacks, the PFC is off-line and the person feels as though they are reliving the trauma. There is little to no access to problem-solving or decision-making capacities that reside in the PFC.

Hippocampus

This structure, part of the limbic system, is involved in memory encoding and the synthesis of experience.

Polyvagal Theory

Porges' (2011) Polyvagal Theory (PVT) has received a lot of attention from attachment researchers, neurobiologists, and professionals who work with traumatized children and youth (and adults). A very simple description of PVT is that Porges discovered an evolutionarily newer myelinated branch of the vagus nerve (the longest nerve in the human body). The PVT, he posits, is associated with physiological characteristics and indicators of social engagement (e.g. the eyes, facial expression, and prosody); thus he named this branch the social engagement system. See Figure 1.5 for a simplified overview of PVT. The theory itself is quite complicated so I invite you to refer to Porges' writings listed in the Reference section.

Moving Toward a More Accurate Description of Trauma's Impact on Children and Youth – Developmental Trauma Disorder

Bessel van der Kolk (2005) and colleagues proposed a new diagnostic category to capture the impact of trauma in children and youth. Researchers suggest that treatment of Developmental Trauma Disorder (DTD) focus on six core components: safety, self-regulation, self-reflective information processing,

Table 1.1 Porges' Polyvagal Theory Simplified

Reptiles			*Mammals*
System	Dorsal vagal (unmyelinated branch of parasympathetic)	Sympathetic nervous system	Ventral branch of parasympathetic nervous system (myelinated)
Function(s)	Immobilization, metabolic conservation, shut-down	Mobilization, enhanced actions (fight/flight)	Social engagement
Area/organ target(s)	Internal visceral organs (e.g. stomach, liver) Below diaphragm	Limbs/periphery (legs, arms)	Complex social and attachment behaviors (seen in eyes, facial muscles, vocalizations) Above diaphragm

traumatic experiences integration, relational engagement, and positive affect enhancement (Cook et al., 2005). While this book focuses on the second core component, self-regulation, the interventions are not typically offered in a linear fashion; thus clinicians may touch on the six components throughout the three phases of treatment. For example, the importance of ensuring internal and external safety is monitored over the course of treatment, not just at the beginning, and positive affect enhancement through cultivation of resources and strengths may start when therapy begins.

Brain Scans

Various brain structures and regions may be impacted by childhood trauma and neglect. Perry's (1997) early well-known images of the comparison between a severely deprived three year old's brain scan and that of a healthy three year old show abnormal development of the cortex and overall smaller size. Since then, there has been an abundance of research documenting the impact of childhood trauma on brain development.

2   Frameworks and Models

The mind is like the wind and the body like the sand: if you want to know how the wind is blowing, you can look at the sand.

(Bonnie Bainbridge Cohen, 2012, p. 1)

This chapter outlines key components of the somatic models and frameworks that inform my work with traumatized youth and their families. The natural utility of somatic methods is reflected in Bainbridge Cohen's eloquent opening quote. A similar structure will be provided for each model or framework: overview, main components, and case illustrations. One question you might be pondering now is the use of framework versus model, so we shall address this up-front. Note that the term *approach* is often used interchangeably with framework. Sometimes it is simply a matter of semantics. For our purposes, we can consider a framework or approach (e.g. ARC, SP) as comprehensive, often comprising models (e.g. the modulation model, the information processing model). Models tend to be more structured and are sometimes manualized (e.g. TF-CBT). There are many other models and frameworks, such as Bainbridge Cohen's Body–Mind Centering, Perry's NMT (Neurosequential Model of Therapeutics) and Gomez-Perales' Attachment-Focused Trauma Treatment for Children and Adolescents, but these are the approaches that I have been trained in and use in my clinical work.

Attachment, Self-Regulation, and Competency (ARC)

Overview

ARC (Attachment, Self-Regulation, and Competency) is a component-based framework that comprises ten core building blocks. The framework is grounded in attachment theory, the impact of traumatic stress, child development, and factors promoting resilience. The latter point is important since strengths and resilience are essential to our work, and often overlooked by clinicians. The ARC manual was developed by Margaret Blaustein and Kristine Kinneburgh of the Justice Resource Institute (JRI) to address complexly traumatized youth (Blaustein & Kinneburgh, 2010). The building blocks are structured in a sequential manner to reflect developmental needs; however, clinicians may find that interventions are not delivered in a linear manner, and they may return to previously addressed skills over the course of treatment. As noted in Chapter 1, repetition is key in forming new neural patterns. ARC is not a short-term intervention: it addresses trauma on individual, family, and systems levels, with the number of sessions ranging from 12 to more than 50 (National Child Traumatic Stress Network, 2012). Since the ARC manual was published in 2010, there have been numerous studies contributing to its ever-increasing evidence base (Arvidson et al., 2011; Hodgdon et al., 2015). Clinical research has demonstrated ARC's effectiveness in reducing PTSD symptoms in males and females, residential school settings, post-adoptive families, and various cultural groups. The JRI offers two-day workshops that highlight the essential pieces of the framework while modeling the playful approach that ARC embodies. Ongoing consultation following the two-day training is recommended.

Main Components of ARC – the Building Blocks

A key feature of ARC is the inclusion of caregiver applications and teaching points throughout the manual. Additionally, ARC offers individual, class-room, group, and milieu adaptations. For each building block, fundamental concepts, teaching points, activities that target specific areas (e.g. recogni-tion of triggers, body awareness), caregiver suggestions, and developmental considerations are expounded. Following is a brief overview of the ten core building blocks.

The three primary domains addressed through the building blocks are: Attachment, Self-Regulation and Competency. A fourth domain, Trauma Experience Integration, culls from and integrates skills covered in the first three domains. Figure 2.1 depicts an image of the ARC block construction, and there now follows a description of the components within the rows.

Bottom Row: Attachment

The Attachment domain includes building blocks for:

a. Caregiver management of affect – in order for caregivers to effectively co-regulate their children, they must be able to regulate themselves.
b. Attunement – the capacity to recognize and respond to the needs of their children is essential to optimal development.
c. Consistent response – children require consistency and predictability. A caregiver's consistent response to various expressions fosters a felt sense of safety.
d. Routines and rituals – reliability and predictability in the form of routines and rituals enhances the child's sense of safety and trust in self and others.

Working with complexly traumatized youth often involves working with intergenerational trauma. Caregivers may not have the skills to regulate themselves,

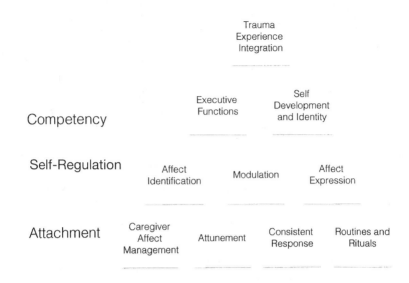

Figure 2.1 ARC (Attachment, Self-Regulation, and Competency) Core Building Blocks
Source: Adapted from Blaustein, M. & Kinneburgh, K. (2010). *Treating Traumatic Stress in Children and Adolescents.* New York: Guilford Press. Used with Permission.

lack the capacity to attune to their child, and may be unable to set clear routines and boundaries. Some caregivers benefit from psychoeducation about developmental expectations, the importance of consistency in response and routines, as well as ways to manage their own affect. The clinician may serve as a co-regulator, and then go on to model interactive regulation during this portion of treatment.

Second Row: Self-Regulation

a. Affect identification – the ability to recognize and differentiate a range of emotions as well as the internal experience of emotion.
b. Modulation – develop the capacity to monitor and regulate one's emotions and internal responses; increase skills to maintain optimal arousal.
c. Affect expression – develop ability to express what one is feeling to effectively have needs met.

    As noted earlier, this book focuses on the second row of ARC's building blocks; thus these concepts will be expanded upon throughout future chapters. Given financial and time constraints, and the absence of a safe attachment figure to participate in treatment, safety and stabilization may be the only phase of trauma treatment addressed with some clients. Within these building blocks, strategies are introduced to assist youth with recognition and management of emotions, physiological states, and "to safely and effectively express internal experience" (Blaustein & Kinneburgh, 2010, p. 39). The ARC framework's manual presents an excellent array of activities and tools for practitioners to develop these capacities in youth.

Third Row: Competency

a. Executive functions – housed in the prefrontal cortex, executive functions include problem-solving skills and delayed responses or inhibition. The prefrontal cortex is often not accessed in traumatized youth who have grown accustomed to living in their limbic system.
b. Self-development and identity – develops over the course of one's lifetime, includes an understanding of self as separate from others and the abilities to see the self as a positive and integrated being.

Finally, the Trauma Experience Integration block sits atop the pyramid. This piece of work strives to address the intrusive memories and related thoughts, somatic experiences, feelings, and beliefs about self and others, and to integrate the skills covered in the three core domains to facilitate the youth's movement toward a coherent sense of self living in the present.

Sensory Motor Arousal Regulation Treatment (SMART)

Overview

SMART integrates theory and foundational skills from trauma theory, sensory integration, occupational therapy, child development, and Sensorimotor Psychotherapy™. Research has provided empirical support for SMART's effectiveness in treating traumatized youth in residential settings (Warner et al., 2013; Warner et al., 2014). There are five core skills used by the SMART therapist:

1. attunement – being aware of, and effectively responding to, youth needs;
2. tracking – monitoring the moment-by-moment experience of the youth;
3. making contact – using words and/or gestures to acknowledge the youth's unfolding experience;
4. therapist as co-regulator – using qualities such as prosody, movement, and activity levels, the therapist works to widen the child's capacity to regulate;
5. mindfulness – therapists assist youth to engage in mindful curiosity of the present moment (i.e. tracking or monitoring), thus the youth engages the prefrontal cortex that is otherwise off-line in dysregulated states.

Through use of the core skills, the SMART therapist works with the youth and caregiver to identify the ways that trauma has impacted the child's emotional and cognitive development, as well as the ways trauma is held and expressed through the body. As a somatic model, SMART recognizes that trauma is stored in the body and expressed through the autonomic nervous system. The child may present in states of high activation (hyperarousal) or extremely low activation (hypoarousal), or may vacillate between states with a biphasic presentation. Since stabilization of the arousal is a prerequisite for trauma processing, the capacity to regulate must be addressed at the beginning of treatment. SMART works with the nervous system in many ways to help children modulate their arousal, including vestibular, proprioception, rhythm, and tactile, frequently combining methods.

A youth's inability to self-regulate negatively impacts the ability to function (and develop) cognitively, emotionally, and behaviorally. At the beginning of treatment, it is helpful to provide caregivers with descriptions of the child's way of thinking, feeling, and doing in dysregulated states. I use a laminated chart to show caregivers how hypoarousal or hyperarousal, as well as a regulated state, may appear in their child across the domains. Caregivers can then begin tracking for signs of dysregulation and use skills, such as co-regulation through prosody or rhythm, to bring their child back into their window of tolerance. The window of tolerance is usually quite narrow when therapy begins, and both therapist and caregiver work with the child to widen their windows over time.

Sensorimotor Psychotherapy™

> Traumatized clients are haunted by the return of trauma-related sensorimotor reactions in such forms as intrusive images, sounds, smells, body sensations, physical pain, constriction, numbing, and the inability to regulate arousal.
>
> (Ogden et al., 2005)

Overview

Sensorimotor Psychotherapy™ (SP), developed by Pat Ogden, is a body-based approach to working with developmental/attachment injuries and trauma. Drawn from the Hakomi method (developed by Ron Kurtz in the 1970s), this framework approaches psychotherapy with the following foundational principles in mind:

1. Mind–body–spirit holism – the therapist works with the mind and body concurrently to explore core beliefs that were created through earlier experiences.
2. Unity – people are composed of parts that make up a whole, living in relation to other systems such as family, cultures, and society.
3. Mindfulness/presence – being fully present in the present moment such that one is able to observe thoughts, feelings, and sensations as they unfold.
4. Nonviolence – SP is a collaborative approach wherein the therapist works to provide a safe environment, moving at the client's pace.

5. Organicity – SP works with the entire system as a whole, encouraging trust in the wisdom of the body as a self-correcting system that naturally strives toward wholeness and homeostasis.

SP's principles contribute to a therapeutic relationship that is respectful, moves at the client's pace, and honors the inherent wisdom of the client's whole self. The therapist models curiosity and compassion while working with the client to uncover core beliefs that are reflected in patterned responses, including gestures, movement, and posture. Psychoeducation, provided up front and throughout the therapeutic process, is a fundamental component in SP work. Psychoeducation aims to impart an understanding of the legacy of trauma on the body, as well as the neurobiological underpinnings of trauma. Furthermore, explaining how working with the body increases the possibility of reaching therapy goals instills hope for change. Therapists often model movement with their own bodies as they are demonstrating the potential for the body to "tell the story" beyond words. Through validation of the client's distressing symptoms as products of early childhood experiences, and appreciation for the ways that these patterns and responses helped the child survive overwhelming experiences, clients feel understood, relieved, and hopeful.

Clients' existing resources are explored (e.g. creative, social, and physical activities used to up or down regulate) and new resources are added as treatment progresses. Resources are essential as clients may find it necessary to ground, center, or contain while moving through the phases of treatment. Clients are encouraged to develop compassion for the emotions and experiences that they may have learned to disown. For example, if being vulnerable was met with disdain or punishment in a child's family of origin, he learns to dismiss or squelch feelings or behaviors that might suggest need. If a child learns that autonomy and independence are not acceptable, she may develop patterns of pleasing others and putting her own needs aside in order to stay in relationship with others (i.e. the primary caregiver). Traumatic experiences, especially those from childhood when the brain is developing, are often stored preverbally and as fragments inaccessible to conscious awareness. These implicit memories may be images, thoughts, feelings, sensations, or impulses.

The body is used as the entry point in SP as the therapist explores the building blocks of experience: cognition, emotions, 5-sense perception, sensations, and movements that have shaped and continue to impact client experiences (Ogden & Minton, 2000). Bromberg (2006) stressed the importance of the therapist working in a way that is "safe but not too safe": working at the edges of the client's window of tolerance to evoke activation but not send them into a state of collapse, dissociation, or hyperarousal. Siegel coined the term "Window of Tolerance" (WOT) to describe the range of arousal that allows us to manage emotions and function optimally (Siegel, 1999). Most significantly, by working at the edge of the window, clients do not have to relive their trauma by going through the details. With sufficient activation, while tracking the client's building blocks of experience moment by moment, the therapist guides the client toward deepening their present moment experience. Beyond insight, this deepening of awareness facilitates change in the building blocks.

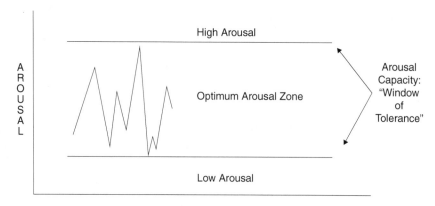

Figure 2.2 The Modulation Model
Source: Ogden, P. & Minton, K. (2000). Sensorimotor Psychotherapy: one method for processing traumatic memory. In *Traumatology*, Vol. VI, 3(3), 1–20. Used with Permission.
* Window of Tolerance: Siegel, D. (1999). *The Developing Mind: Toward a Neurobiology of Interpersonal Experience*. New York: Guilford Press.

Like many therapeutic approaches, SP is phase-oriented, which means there is a focus on safety and stabilization (phase one) when treatment begins. There are also five stages in a typical therapy session. In SP the five stages of the process are:

C	Container
A	Accessing
P	Processing
T	Transformation
I	Integration

"The stages add structure and support for the flow of the session, help to ensure that therapist and client work in manageable chunks, and guide the use of therapeutic skills" (Sharpe-Lohrasbe, personal communication). A session can move through all five stages in a therapy hour, allowing the client to experience either minor or major transformations in her way of moving through the world, her self-concept or core beliefs, or to reinstate an act of defense. The reinstatement of an act of defense, such as fleeing an overwhelming situation or setting a boundary when it was impossible to do so at the time of the trauma, is extremely profound and empowering for clients.

Main Components of SP

The SP therapist utilizes a set of skills to help clients explore and change patterned responses that no longer serve a purpose. SP core skills are:

1) tracking;
2) contact statements;
3) framing present moment experience through the building blocks of experience (also known as core organizers);
4) mindfulness questions and mindful directives;
5) mindful experiments.

Adaptations to SP for Youth and Case Illustration

Children and youth are naturally curious; these qualities make SP a great fit for working with traumatized youth:

1) play and experiments – encourages creativity and curiosity;
2) movement – difficult for youth, especially younger children, to sit for an hour;
3) beyond words – younger children have not yet developed the ability vis-à-vis brain development to effectively express themselves through words, and youth often lack the vocabulary and life experience to accurately articulate what they are feeling and experiencing.

Caregiver involvement is encouraged throughout treatment. Not only is the caregiver a consistent resource; they also play a role in enhancing youth's capacity for self-regulation. Caregiver as interactive regulator is covered extensively in Chapter 7.

Case Illustration

Vincent

We were introduced to Vincent earlier. As described, Vincent's physical presentation vacillated between absolute stillness and agitation. Vincent possessed fair body awareness, he was articulate and forthcoming, and he was motivated to work through his traumatic experiences. He was also curious and creative; such qualities lend themselves to Sensorimotor Psychotherapy™ (SP). Following a comprehensive assessment, Vincent and I began exploring, enhancing, and developing resources. Resources in SP can be internal, an innate capacity such as intelligence, or external, such as access to a supportive family and social network (Ogden & Fisher, 2015). Resources can also be categorized as survival or creative. Survival resources are those developed and used to cope with the trauma, such as dissociation, self-injury, or substance abuse, and continue as maladaptive patterns beyond the trauma. Creative resources are capacities or skills that enable one to feel connected to the self and others, and to function well in the world. Vincent's existing resources included intelligence, biking, running, swimming, and creativity (music, art).

Following the traumatic experiences, Vincent lost interest in art and physical activity, except biking when he needed to "blow off steam," and he withdrew from family and friends. After taking stock of existing resources, we discussed ways to enhance other areas such as nature, and to reactivate his interest in arts and social activity. Simultaneously, we worked on expanding his window of tolerance through the following:

1. Psychoeducation about the window of tolerance and development of tracking skills – increased awareness of the upper and lower edges of his window of tolerance, expanding his window, and developing skills to track and bring himself back into his window. To help Vincent track his somatic experience, a "menu" of sensory words was provided and he was asked to consider his physiological experience in various situations between sessions. Vincent was keen to increase his awareness and ability to track his somatic experience, and he reported that he kept the list in a pocket much of the time in the early stages of treatment.
2. Grounding – pushing his feet into the floor, feeling the support of the earth beneath him.
3. Containment – pressing into the wall with his arms, as well as tapping along his edges (e.g. arms, legs). Vincent found the latter technique particularly helpful and used it to bring himself back when triggered into a flashback throughout the treatment process. He noticed that, with practice, he was able to bring himself back more quickly and the flashbacks diminished in intensity over time.
4. Centering – Vincent was taught to attend to his breath, expand the breath into his abdomen, and place one hand on his heart while the other rested on his stomach. Vincent was invited to imagine a healing color filling his abdominal cavity with each inhalation. Vincent found this quite calming and continued to practice it for years (we worked together for three years).

Another area we addressed was boundaries. When Vincent was first asked to form a boundary with yarn, he wrapped the yarn around his body. Subsequent discussions revealed that he felt he could not protect himself and that he had difficulty recognizing his needs as separate from others. We experimented with ways that Vincent could feel safe, such as setting nonverbal boundaries. Note that Vincent was also dealing with body image issues and eating-disordered behavior, I was careful not to use the word "body" lest he be triggered. Instead we referred to "what's happening inside," for example. Vincent was experiencing a great deal of shame and self-loathing as well (this work is detailed later in Chapter 12). Over time, Vincent learned what felt right for him in terms of physical and psychological boundaries, and he learned to recognize and express his own needs.

Sequencing is an SP intervention aimed at recalibrating trauma-related sympathetic arousal (Ogden & Fisher, 2015). Through mindful tracking of the body's involuntary movements, such as trembling or shaking, the client is able to discharge the energy that has been stored from the trauma. Vincent was able to engage in sequencing only after he was capable of tracking and managing dysregulation, his window of tolerance was expanded, and he trusted the wisdom of his body. He had knowledge of the building blocks of experience and had developed the ability to distinguish them and to use them in service of regulating arousal. SP's building blocks of present experience are: 5-sense perception, thoughts, emotions, movement, and sensations (Ogden, Minton & Pain, 2006). We had engaged in many experiments over a period of about two years, often employing playfulness and expressive arts, including reinstating acts of defense (Ogden, Goldstein & Fisher, 2012) while working with slivers of memories prior to sequencing. Vincent had demonstrated the capacity for mindful awareness and tracking his somatic experience. A sliver of memory is sufficient to enable trauma work at the edges of the window of tolerance without causing retraumatization. Following is a brief example of sequencing:

> After a period of discussion and agreement about what to work on this session, I invite Vincent to begin talking about the incident at the bathhouse. He is reminded that he can stop at any time that he feels overwhelmed. Therapist tracks and makes contact with contraction-like movements in Vincent's stomach area. These movements had been observed previously when Vincent was distressed, and we had discussed their presence and ways to calm his autonomic system at these times.

K: When you see yourself in that room, what happens in your body?

V: I feel scared.

K: Yes, I can imagine how scary it was. And how do you notice that fear in your body?

V: Um, yeah, I see the guys' hands reaching for me.

K: You see the guys' hands. Notice what is happening inside when you see the guys' hands? *(Client is redirected to his body sensations, using a directed mindfulness question, as we continue to move through arousal while maintaining the mindful awareness that keeps the prefrontal cortex engaged.)*

V: I notice my stomach gets tight, it feels like it's quivery.

K: Uh huh, your stomach is quivery. Just stay with that quivery sensation, Vincent, and notice what happens next with the quivering.

V: It feels more quivery, like bigger waves, and I feel it in my chest too.

K: Let's stay with that quivering. *(Vincent's involuntary movements are spreading and more intense. There is observable shaking in his upper chest and shoulders. I check in with him to ensure he is still present, not overwhelmed or outside his window of tolerance. After a period of shaking, I make contact with my observations.)* The shaking seems to be spreading, eh?

V: Yeah, it's um, well, weird. *(Vincent's eyes are closed as he finds it easier to drop into his body and be mindful with his eyes closed. His affect appears somewhat distressed at this point, with subtle eye and mouth twitching.)*

K: Yes, your body knows what it needs to do, just let it happen.

V: Okay. *(Vincent continues to shake throughout his abdominal and chest areas, with some twitching in his legs and arms. After 30 seconds or so, the shaking appears to slow down.)*

K: What's happening with the quivering now, Vincent, or what wants to happen?

V: Well, it's not so strong, it's smaller waves.

K: Uh huh, notice that the quivering is easing off. Let's stay with that. *(The movements settle, Vincent's body appears to relax, and he has a slight grin.)* What do you notice now with the quivering?

V: It's almost stopped, like I don't feel the quivering all over. It's really weird to watch this in myself.

K: Yes, it's pretty cool how the shaking that needs to happen just happens, eh?

V: Yeah. *(Vincent takes a deep sigh and slowly opens his eyes. His lips form a slight smile again, then his eyebrows form an inquisitive expression. He takes another deep breath and nods.)*

K: How are you doing, Vincent?

V: I feel okay. Yeah, I feel okay. *(We take a few minutes to allow Vincent to integrate his experience, to reflect on the movements as his body releases energy related to the trauma. Note that we had another session with sequencing, with similar sensorimotor responses evoked by other building blocks of his experience.)*

After the sequencing sessions, Vincent reported feeling safer and more confident in his body, that he was triggered less easily by reminders of his traumatic experiences, and that he was more capable of being affectionate with his boyfriend. He was visibly less tense, and the appearance of a freeze response (activation coupled with immobilization) markedly diminished.

Somatic Experiencing® (SE)

By Michelle Dick, C. Psych. Associate

Overview of Somatic Experiencing®

Somatic Experiencing® is a psychobiological approach to treating the impact of traumatic experiences that is guided by an understanding of trauma physiology. This includes an understanding of how the body responds to and is affected by experiences that are traumatic, as well as what supports healthy nervous system functioning. Somatic Experiencing® is the evolution of Dr. Peter A. Levine's life work based on his multidisciplinary studies and clinical work in medical biophysics and psychology (Somatic Experiencing® Trauma Institute, 2013). Dr. Levine first developed this method in the 1970s in the context of his clinical work with survivors of shock trauma, for example automobile accidents, surgery, assaults, war, and natural disasters (Levine, 1997). Since that time Dr. Levine has continued to develop and refine this approach, creating a psychobiological treatment framework that informs work across a range of traumatic impacts including complex trauma, early trauma, attachment trauma, and ongoing stress and trauma, in addition to shock trauma. In his book *Waking the Tiger* Dr. Levine shares that he "does not view post-traumatic stress disorder (PTSD) as pathology to be managed, suppressed, or adjusted to, but the result of a natural process gone awry" (Levine, 1997, p. 3). From this perspective, the therapeutic approach of Somatic Experiencing® addresses the nonverbal, biologically driven aspects of trauma and focuses on supporting normative somatic responses and processes. This involves recognizing instinctual survival responses and supporting the autonomic nervous system to move toward increasing organization, regulation, and resilience (Somatic Experiencing® Trauma Institute, 2013).

Main Components of Somatic Experiencing®

In Somatic Experiencing® sessions the emphasis is shifted away from the narrative of the traumatic event, and instead careful attention to inner sensations and subtle movements are central to the therapeutic work. The focus remains in the here and now with attention directed to the felt sense as it emerges in the present moment. While sessions may be conversational, the therapeutic work and pacing of the session is guided by what is happening at a physiological level, within the autonomic nervous system, as sensed by the client and observed by the therapist. Tuning into the inner sensations that accompany the body's natural rhythm of pendulation between contraction and expansion helps to create the conditions for finding stability and calm within the autonomic nervous system, while also exploring distress in a gradual way that is not overwhelming. In this way, it becomes possible to access and work with the instinctual threat-response reactions that continue to loop within an individual's nervous system, and to support shifts in physiological, nervous system processes that occur beneath the level of conscious awareness or explicit verbal memory. Integration across other aspects of functioning, for example thoughts, memories, emotions, and actions, also becomes available as new patterns within the nervous system are supported.

The following case illustrations are shared as examples of how Somatic Experiencing® can inform work with children. These case illustrations are based on this writer's experience of working with children; however, they have been fictionalized to maintain confidentiality.

Sophie

Sophie was a 9-year-old girl whose mother brought her in because anxiety was increasingly affecting Sophie's life. They reported that they first noticed the anxiety two years ago, when Sophie was 7 years old. Sophie's mother identified an event that she felt changed something for Sophie and contributed to the development of the anxiety. She shared that approximately two years ago she and Sophie were at the mall together shopping in a children's store that Sophie was very familiar with. As they shopped, Sophie's mother kept Sophie in her sight. Just as Sophie stopped to admire a toy that caught her eye, there was a loud disturbance in the hallway of the mall. Sophie was startled and when she looked up to find her mother, Sophie could not see her. Sophie did not realize that her mother was nearby and had Sophie in her sight.

Since Sophie's mother identified this event, and the timing fit with the development of the anxiety, we made a plan to start by specifically working with this event. The writer suggested working from a somatic perspective and, after talking about why and what that might be like, Sophie's mother agreed and we scheduled a session.

When Sophie and her mother arrived for the session, Sophie smiled shyly and stayed close by her mother's side. At first we took time to just visit with a view to connecting and settling. After about ten minutes and when Sophie appeared more comfortable, we started by talking just a little about the day of the mall event that Sophie's mother had already shared. As we talked, Sophie's face became tense, her lips were pulled together, her gaze moved around the room, and she started shifting in her chair. The writer took this opportunity to notice how scary talking about this experience was for Sophie, and to normalize how of course it would have been scary. Sophie's mother agreed and we spent a short amount of time talking about that. Then, with the intention of supporting stability and calm within Sophie's nervous system, the writer asked Sophie if it would be possible for her to imagine that day at the mall and to imagine that when she looked up to find her mom, she saw her mom. Sophie shook her head yes and the writer encouraged her to take her time imagining. After a little while it was apparent that Sophie's body was settling, her muscles noticeably relaxed, and a small smile came to her mouth. The writer commented that this seemed different and asked Sophie if it felt different in her body. Sophie answered that yes, it did. After a little while Sophie's mother started talking about how scary it must have been and how sorry she was. In response to this Sophie looked at her mom and smiled and then her face and body appeared to tense a little again. At this point the writer asked Sophie if she would be okay with trying more imagining and, with the intention of supporting a little more activation, asked Sophie if she could imagine her mother being farther away but still where Sophie could see her. At this Sophie started squirming in her chair, she appeared very tense, and she shook her head no. In an effort to attune with Sophie the writer said okay, yes, that's too much isn't it. And Sophie agreed. Then the writer asked Sophie if it would be possible to change anything on that day, what would have helped Sophie the most on that day. Sophie looked over at her mom and said it would have been to have a plan that even if she couldn't see her mother, that she would know where to find her mother in the store. The writer asked Sophie if she could notice how her body felt now and she paused to notice. For a moment there was a softening in her face and body, a settling, and then a great deal of movement and squirming emerged and big tears welled up in Sophie's eyes. With the hope of supporting this activation to find a successful completion the writer encouraged Sophie to do what she wanted to do now. In response to this encouragement Sophie immediately got up and went to her mother, curling up in her mother's arms like a much younger child might. Sophie's mother held her and comforted her. After a while Sophie relaxed, she appeared calm, color came into her cheeks, a sparkle came into her eyes, and there was a sense of ease and happiness about her. As they walked out, after we said goodbye, there was a spring in Sophie's step that had not been there before, and she still looked happy with color in her cheeks and a sparkle in her eye.

George

George was a 7-year-old boy whose parents brought him in for help with the sadness and distress of learning that his grandfather, who had lived with the family since George was born, had a terminal illness. George's parents shared that he loved spending time with his grandfather, who had, over the years, become one of George's primary caretakers. George and his family were already acquainted with the writer from doing some work together in the past. At this time, since George's parents were not able to attend sessions, we made a plan for George to meet with the writer on a weekly basis, while the writer also kept in close contact with his parents by telephone. George's parents reported that since receiving this sad news George was noticeably more hyperactive, easily upset, and very tearful. They also shared that the difficulties extended to school and peer relationships, and that George was consistently coming home from school in tears, feeling left out.

When George arrived for sessions, he often seemed full of energy and greeted the writer with a lot of bouncing and excited talking about what we could do during our time together. We developed a routine of spending some time together in that high-energy state at the beginning of each session and then, when George appeared to settle a little, we practiced a somatic exercise that involved pretending to be a tree. The writer introduced this activity with the intention of supporting some stability and calm to emerge within George's experience at a physiological level. George enjoyed this exercise and spontaneously used it in ways that appeared to support his nervous system. We always practiced it together, feeling our feet on the ground, imagining the feeling of roots going down into the ground, and noticing the feeling of a trunk, branches, and leaves. The writer encouraged George to let himself notice what this felt like in his body. All on his own George would shake his arms, hands, and fingers, pretending to be a tree blowing in the wind. He would also often spontaneously act out cycles of winter and summer, death and rebirth. As we practiced and imagined this together, there was a noticeable settling in George's demeanor and body. While the energy remained, his movements appeared softer and slightly slowed down, his breathing became deeper and more relaxed, and he often paused and made lingering but comfortable eye contact with the writer. Following this, George would ask to play with the dollhouse, and he tended to explore themes of family, togetherness, crisis, loss, death, helping each other, and making it through difficult times. As experienced by the writer, practicing this somatic activity consistently appeared to help ground the session and support shifts in George's nervous system that allowed the processing through play to be more accessible.

Bibliography

Levine, P.A. (1997). *Waking the Tiger: Healing Trauma*. Berkeley, CA: North Atlantic Books.

Levine, P.A. (2010). *In an Unspoken Voice: How the Body Releases Trauma and Restores Goodness*. Berkeley, CA: North Atlantic Books.

Levine, P.A. (2015). *Trauma and Memory: Brain and Body in a Search for the Living Past* [Kindle version]. Retrieved from www.amazon.com

Levine, P.A. & Kline, M. (2007). *Trauma Through a Child's Eyes: Awakening the Ordinary Miracle of Healing*. Berkeley, CA: North Atlantic Books; Lyons, CO: ERGOS Institute Press.

Payne P., Levine, P.A. & Crane-Godreau, M.A. (2015). Somatic Experiencing: Using Interoception and Proprioception as Core Elements of Trauma Therapy. *Frontiers in Psychology: Consciousness Research*. 6(93). Retrieved from https://traumahealing.org/resources/

Somatic Experiencing® Trauma Institute (2013). *SE Professional Training* [training brochure/booklet]. Boulder, CO: Somatic Experiencing® Trauma Institute.

Taylor, P.J., Ph.D., SEP, CGP, FAGPA, & Saint-Laurent, R., Psy.D., SEP, CGP (2017). Group Psychotherapy Informed by the Principles of Somatic Experiencing: Moving Beyond Trauma to Embodied Relationship. *International Journal of Group Psychotherapy*. 67:sup.1, S171–S181. Retrieved from https://traumahealing.org/resources/

Blending SP and Trauma Focused Cognitive Behavioral Therapy

Overview of TF-CBT

Trauma Focused Cognitive Behavioral Therapy (TF-CBT) is an evidence-based practice developed in the 1990s by Judith Cohen, Esther Deblinger, and Anthony Mannarino. The model was originally developed to treat sexually abused youth. Since then, extant research supports the efficacy of TF-CBT to treat children exhibiting symptoms of PTSD from exposure to a range of adverse experiences including domestic violence, war and terrorism, and traumatic grief (Cary & McMillen, 2012; Jensen et al., 2014; Mannarino et al., 2012; Ramirez de Arellano et al., 2014). Furthermore, follow-up assessment demonstrates retention of improvement over time (Konanur et al., 2015; Mannarino et al., 2012). TF-CBT is a structured, manualized, and directive approach and thus is not an approach that feels comfortable for all clinicians. Given its structure and expected timeframe, TF-CBT may not be a fit for some populations (e.g. dissociative youth, youth with cognitive limitations) and might not be the best approach for youth with complex trauma histories. Recent research on the use of TF-CBT with adolescents with complex trauma (Cohen et al., 2012) demonstrates that the model may be effective when treatment length is extended (e.g. up to 25 sessions). Research on the use of TF-CBT within three months of a traumatic event highlights the importance of early intervention (e.g. Roberts, 2009).

Main Components of TF-CBT

TF-CBT is typically delivered in 12–16 sessions and follows a sequence divided into thirds, all sessions providing gradual exposure to the traumatic event. Gradual exposure is intended to desensitize the child as preparation for the Trauma Narrative. An integral feature of TF-CBT is inclusion of a parent or supportive caregiver throughout the process. Caregivers are provided with opportunities to hear how the child is doing after each session, receive information about the impact of trauma, and learn parenting strategies that might be helpful with the behavioral manifestations of their child's trauma. While this is not always possible, the inclusion of a caregiver provides opportunity for the youth to reinforce skills outside the clinical setting, and caregivers are given strategies to best support the child throughout the treatment process.

Prior to implementing treatment, youth are administered a battery of tests. The same tools are administered post-treatment to capture the treatment effect and to determine if additional treatment is required. Commonly used measures include the TSCC, TSCYC, CBCL, UCLA-PTSD, MASC, and CDI. (Note: These measures are described in Chapter 3.)

The acronym PRACTICE is used for the eight components of TF-CBT, broken into thirds over the course of treatment:

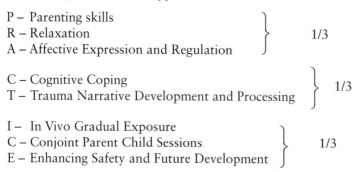

P – Parenting skills
R – Relaxation   } 1/3
A – Affective Expression and Regulation

C – Cognitive Coping
T – Trauma Narrative Development and Processing   } 1/3

I – In Vivo Gradual Exposure
C – Conjoint Parent Child Sessions   } 1/3
E – Enhancing Safety and Future Development

Brief Description of the Components

Psychoeducation/Parenting skills involve providing the child and caregiver with information about trauma and the potential impact. This offers validation and normalization, reducing the child's and caregiver's anxieties and fears about the child being abnormal because of the abuse or never being able to move beyond the abuse. Additionally, this piece of work includes parenting skills, tailored to meet the specific needs of that caregiver, to effectively manage emotional and behavioral consequences of the abuse. For example, the therapist might suggest development of predictability and consistency via bedtime routines. Therapists also work with caregivers, through modeling and psychoeducation, to ensure they are prepared for the Trauma Narrative that may be shared with them later in treatment (Ramirez de Arellano et al., 2014).

Relaxation – Children, and caregivers, are taught relaxation and stress management skills, often using games, play, or expressive arts methods. Interventions are selected based on the child's interests and strengths. For example, some children like to read books (e.g. *Peaceful Piggy Meditation* might be used). Others respond better to audio or visual stimuli so these features would be integrated into interventions. Blending Sensorimotor Psychotherapy™ (SP) into this component expands the possibilities and increases the playfulness and creativity of the work.

Affective Expression and Regulation – Children, and caregivers, are educated about the range of emotions, the importance of expressing emotions effectively, and how to regulate their emotions. Games, such as feeling words charades with the child or including the caregiver, are fun ways to engage youth in this process. Assisting youth to understand the difference between a feeling (emotion) and a sensation, and to recognize the physiological precursors to experiencing an emotion, is a benefit of adding SP to this component.

Cognitive Coping – This component of TF-CBT brings in the cognitive triangle and thought-stopping practices. Again, drawing from the youth's particular interests and skills, a therapist can be creative and make difficult processes less onerous for young clients. There is plenty of opportunity to include children's natural curiosity, a core feature of SP, in this component.

Trauma Narrative (TN) – The TN represents the middle third of TF-CBT. It can take four to six sessions, depending on the level of detail provided by the child, how able she is to identify and express her thoughts and feelings related to the trauma, and how resourced she is. Depending on the aforementioned factors, the clinician may have to pause and return to previous components (relaxation, etc.). The TN can be created in the form of a story, a dance, or a theatre performance, or can be represented with images. Younger children many choose to use toys or puppets to tell their TN. Features of SP are not added here since SP works with a sliver of the memory rather than the details.

In vivo Gradual Exposure – Desensitization, which occurs during the completion of the TN.

Conjoint Sessions – Conjoint sessions are an integral part of TF-CBT. Clinicians meet with the caregiver and child after the individual session to review material covered during the session. This offers opportunity for the caregiver to provide positive feedback, for the child to demonstrate newly acquired skills, and to plan routines or activities that will help the child at home.

Enhancing Safety and Future Development – While this is considered the final component of treatment, I tend to integrate strategies throughout the course of treatment. The goal here is to provide strategies (e.g. assertiveness) and knowledge (e.g. healthy sexuality) that will benefit the child and hopefully return him to his developmental trajectory.

Case Illustration

Dylan

Dylan was 7 years old when he was referred to a children's mental health agency by local child protection services. He was identified as having difficulties in school related to inattention, aggression with peers, and he had a history of being sexually abused by an older male cousin. One of his mother's biggest concerns was Dylan's refusal to use the washroom at school, tendency to squat "like a frog" on the toilet rather than sit, and frequent constipation because he avoided elimination for as long as he could. Dylan presented with extremely high activity and arousal levels (hyperarousal) so I knew from the beginning of treatment that interventions had to be creative and active with this youngster.

The first third of the TF-CBT model addresses parent education, coping skills (for child and caregiver), and enhancing affect recognition and expression. Dylan liked to draw and he loved sports. Meeting Dylan where he was energy-wise was important to maintaining interest and engagement in treatment. For relaxation and coping skills, I included go-to interventions such as *Peaceful Piggy Meditation* (MacLean, 2006) and Yoga Pretzels (Guber, 2005). Dylan enjoyed the story and went on to create a space in the corner of his bedroom, with a bell and cushion, where he could sit in stillness. He was also taught to invite the bell, a gentle alternative to striking the bowl with the small wooden mallet, and subsequent sessions were started with the sound of the singing bowl. We made the "mind in a jar," which he loved and kept on his bedside table as a concrete reminder to allow himself to settle in order to see and think clearly. Dylan was not a fan of other strategies such as progressive relaxation. SP was blended in this third of the model with activities to increase mindfulness, such as *Mindful Movements* (Nhat Hahn, 2008), and grounding by pushing his feet into the floor. Dylan giggled during this activity because he liked the idea of pushing his toes through the upper mucky layer to the solid ground beneath. In the parent portion, his mother was taught and practiced similar skills to increase her capacity for self-regulation. Each session ended with Dylan demonstrating his new skill for his mother, thereby enhancing his sense of mastery and competence throughout the course of treatment.

The second third of the model consists of cognitive coping and the trauma narrative (TN) with the notion that the child is being gradually desensitized. Around this time, my agency was undergoing some renovations. I was in my office as I watched a worker remove small orange plastic cones from the ceiling sprinklers. I thought of Dylan, his need for activity, his love of sports, and our upcoming session on the cognitive triangle, so I asked the worker if I might have a few of the orange cones. On the cones, I wrote feelings, behaviors, and thoughts, and referred to them as the ABC pylons, or Running the Bases. We were going to incorporate play and mindfulness into the session. When Dylan came in for his session, we first went over the differences and the relationships between the three. We reviewed examples of each. Dylan was visibly itching to slide down off the couch and onto the floor with the pylons (see Figure 2.3). First, I invited Dylan to take a moment to scan his body and notice whatever there was to notice before we played the game. He had learned this practice previously. I watched as Dylan's chest settled with a slow exhalation and he opened his eyes with a smile. We then began the game where a word was offered, such as "skating" or "sad" or "I'm hungry," and Dylan slid into the base (the pylon that represented that thought, feeling, or behavior). He was thrilled that he got them all correct! Dylan was able to maintain focus and think clearly by allowing his body to move during this activity. We then moved to a more complex cognitive activity with the pylons to help Dylan recognize that he could change his feelings by changing his thoughts. He chose to hop from pylon to pylon for this activity. For example, as he stood at the thinking pylon, we explored alternative thoughts he might have about a situation. He hopped to the feeling pylon when he identified the feeling that might go with each thought. Again, we followed his individual session with a joint parent session so Dylan could demonstrate his new awareness and knowledge.

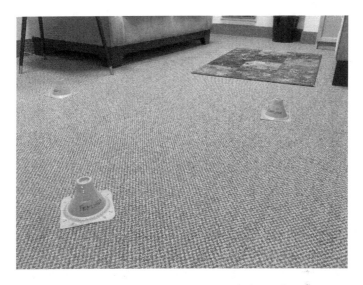

Figure 2.3 Running the Bases: Getting Creative and Physical with TF-CBT

In terms of the TN, Dylan was encouraged to remain present and use his grounding and coping skills as he worked through the story. At the completion of the TN, when he created an alternative ending, we experimented with movements that might lead to the new ending. One time, Dylan noticed that his arms wanted to come up and his hands curled into fists. I encouraged him to slow down the movement and study it. I offered a cushion for him to connect with and he pushed through with his little fists, with frequent reminders to slow down and notice what's happening in his body. He was asked to notice if any sounds wanted to come out, and he responded with a low growl. We engaged in the pushing until Dylan indicated that it was enough for him. Dylan was able to reinstate a mobilizing defensive action, that is, completed a truncated action (i.e. to push away in order to defend himself) that wanted to happen at the time of the trauma. As we finished treatment, Dylan's mother reported that his aggressive behaviors had decreased (but were not eliminated), and teachers reported he could remain seated for longer periods and he was less disruptive in the classroom. Most significant to Dylan and his mother, Dylan was able to sit on the toilet when going to the washroom, and he experienced constipation less frequently. Neurobiologically speaking, Dylan's sympathetic activation decreased and his parasympathetic system activation increased to enable improved functioning of his digestive processes.

Blending SP and EMDR

By Rochelle Sharpe Lohrasbe, PhD

Overview and History of EMDR Therapy

EMDR Therapy, as it is now referred to, was first written about back in the 1980s. Founder Francine Shapiro tells a story describing how she "discovered" EMDR by noticing that moving her eyes while thinking about a troubling circumstance decreased the degree of angst she felt. She published her first write up on the EMD "technique," as it was referred to initially, back in 1987. The first clinical studies on EMDR were published in 1989. Along with CBT, EMDR is one of the most investigated approaches in psychotherapy. A fair proportion of this data has been collected in studies of children and youth in the therapeutic setting.

With more than 40,000 clinicians trained (van der Kolk, 2001), EMDR Therapy has proven to be a flexible and valuable approach for many clients seeking therapy. Adopting a primarily top-down (beliefs, emotions, body) view of overwhelming and/or self-framing experience of the person, EMDR Therapy is adept at tackling a plethora of issues. Efficacy studies have demonstrated the value of the EMDR approach across many diagnoses (OCD, PTSD, ASD, etc.) and several variations of the approach have been used for attachment focused treatment (Adler-Tapia & Settle, 2017; Gomez, 2013; Parnell, 2013; Wesselmann, Schweitzer & Armstrong, 2014). Adler-Tapia & Settle (2017) highlight some research with children and lament the lack.

Adaptive Information Processing (AIP)

Shapiro advanced the notion that, given the right information, people tend toward healing following traumatic incidents. Her work with vets revealed that when bilateral eye movements were paired with the provision of new information or alternate information (to what the person got stuck on at the time of the event), the vets could change beliefs and arrive at new meanings from past experience.

In her own words, Shapiro (2001) describes AIP as "a neurological balance in a distinct physiological system which enables the information to be processed in the perspective of an adaptive processing...Useful information is learned and stored with the appropriate affect and is available for future use."

AIP differs from extinction-based exposure techniques because it relies on the intrinsic capacity of the mind to favor health. Soloman and Shapiro (2008) explain that during an overwhelming event our minds cannot retain a broad view of the experience as we narrow our perceptions to critical aspects necessary for survival. For example, if we are faced with an attacker who wields a weapon, we often become fixated on the weapon in the moment and are unable to include in our awareness other details of the experience. Thus, treatment approaches that focus on exposure might have us reduce our reactions to weapons while we are in the comfort of a safe office environment. The AIP model suggests that if we revisit the memory, we can attend to other details while safe, and that will influence memory reconsolidation. On subsequent recollection, the memory is not as distressing.

Eight Phases of EMDR Therapy

EMDR Therapy (EMDR) comprises eight phases that begin from client intake, preparation, through memory processing, to completion and follow up for the top down – beliefs, then emotions and then the body approach.

Specifically, the eight phases are:

Phase 1: History Taking and Case Conceptualization

Typically, an EMDR history taking centers around significant events relating to limiting beliefs. Often events such as parental separation, the first day of kindergarten, being bullied at school, not being picked for the team, all the way through the witnessing of domestic violence, being molested, surviving a terrorist event, or becoming a refugee, have a profound effect on our beliefs about self, others, and the world in general. Such events become potential *targets* for EMDR processing. It is more interesting to the therapist who uses EMDR to gain an understanding of the meaning the client attached to an event, or the belief they adopted, than to hear all the details of the event (although these will become more important in later phases). Some clients may report one or two very significant events in their lives, while others will have many and complex events to convey.

Phase 2: Preparation

The degree of complexity, the age at which events occurred, and the robustness of resources (internal, external, to keep this simple, when really it isn't) help the therapeutic dyad determine the readiness of the client for subsequent stages. Some clients already have what they need to be able to revisit distressing memories, while others will spend significantly more time in this phase, laying the groundwork for processing to take place. Within the EMDR approach there are several protocols and suggestions for the development of resources for stabilizing and preparing clients to move forward in the process.

Phase 3: Assessment

The use of assessment within the eight-phase approach speaks to the usual way in which targets are identified and brought to present moment recall. EMDR is a top-down approach, so it begins with belief, or thoughts, and includes emotional aspects and also physical aspects of the target in order to "light up" the memory network and associated networks, such as the adaptive networks, prior to moving toward taking the sting out of the memory. Essentially, this brings the client to a state which has them with one foot in the past and one foot in the present so that the event can be reviewed with all the advantages of what is known now (in safety and perhaps with the benefit of maturity) that wasn't known or available to the person back then.

Phase 4: Desensitization

This phase often resembles exposure techniques in that the client runs through all their reactions to the event while in the safety of the therapist's office and in the presence of a safe, caring observer. Eye movements are used during this phase and clients are encouraged to notice what happens as they recall their experience. Metaphors such as watching a movie or riding a train and watching the scenes roll by are often used to keep the progression moving forward. Eye movements or their variations – like taps or auditory clicks – are delivered in sets, and pauses are taken to check in with the client's experience. Often, new insights emerge ("Oh, I didn't realize there was a way out" or "I had to do that to stay safe"), vehement emotions – rage, terror, and panic – move through and the body becomes clear of tensions and distress, returning to a more relaxed open stance. Checking in with the distress and the subjective rating periodically guides the therapist and client through Phase 4.

Phase 5: Installation

This phase approaches the event from another, positive, perspective. We began by identifying a negative belief and now we move toward finding its more positive counterpart by answering the question, "What would you have rather believed about yourself?" In theory, the client shifts from "I'm going to die" to "I survived" or from "I'm a failure" to "I did the best I could and that's good enough." Switching over to the positive perspective might elicit a few more fragments of the memory which need further processing.

Phase 6: Body Scan

EMDR relies heavily on the client's capacity for self-awareness, reflection, and articulation. It mostly accesses memory that is available upon request in the client's memory banks – explicit or autobiographical memory. Seeking the most robust resolution, the body scan is a mechanism that addresses the implicit memory systems where information is held as tensions, heart rate, breathing rate and quality, among other physiological data. By asking the client to scan their body and check for clarity, we have another means to ensure complete processing.

Phase 7: Closure

There are times when the memory banks hold much more information than can be processed during a typical one hour session, so there needs to be a way to bring all this processing to a close and not have the clients leave the office in some altered state. This phase addresses those issues. Frequently clients are informed that now processing has occurred, the client's AIP networks may continue to process the information released during the session. Safety plans, follow up, and a reminder of resources are often discussed to bring the session to close.

Phase 8: Reevaluation

Since processing may continue between sessions, it is important to begin where the client is at when checking in on the events of the previous session. Images may have changed, emotions may have shifted, and beliefs may have undergone revision. Reevaluation allows us to ask, "What is still upsetting about this memory or issue we have been working on?" The client's response takes the session back up into Phase 3, and we repeat. Treatment is not complete until EMDR has focused on the past memories that are contributing to the problem, the present situations that are disturbing, and what skills the client may need for the future.

EMDR *and Sensorimotor Psychotherapy™: Mutually Enhancing*

Integrating the approaches of EMDR Therapy and Sensorimotor Psychotherapy™ (SP) can work well as both fall under the broader category of information processing models. Since youth represent a group with significant variations in developmental stages, the addition of Sensorimotor Psychotherapy™ increases flexibility and provides options for processing that are a better fit to the youth client. Specifically, the information that becomes part of the EMDR Therapy Phase 3 (Assessment of the target) can be obtained from some youth in its usual fashion – top down. However, some youth clients have not yet solidified a strong sense of self or struggle to find the words to accurately articulate their beliefs or, given their overwhelming experience, are unable to identify a single belief for an experience since there are several conflicting, disorganized, or incomplete beliefs which impede their expression. SP, also being concerned with body, emotions, and beliefs, supports flipping of this third phase of EMDR – whereby the clinician can get the belief from the bottom up. Less mental effort, confusion, and risk of shame interfering in the process help keep the set up for processing on track and contained (Sharpe Lohrasbe, 2015).

Consistent with lighting up the neural network (EMDR) and working at the edges of the window of tolerance (Siegel, 1999) as part of the Modulation Model (SP; Ogden, Minton & Pain, 2006), clinicians work in the space that is "safe but not too safe" (SP) or the "zone of optimal arousal" (EMDR). In other words, the client must be in a state of dual attention, capable of having one foot in the past while simultaneously processing the disturbing memory in the safe present situation. By maintaining dual awareness, the client is able to incorporate new information into the reconsolidated memory. This is what Francine Shapiro was referring to when she first used the term Adaptive Information Processing and set this out as a basic premise for EMDR.

At times each of the two approaches offers something complementary to the other. EMDR does not emphasize information at the somatic level, thus potentially missing important and relevant information in children and youth experience. As arousal states reach the upper edges of the person's window of tolerance, and in fact should arousal exceed the child's integrative capacity, somatic resources (alignment, movement, breath, grounding, etc.) are quick modulators of autonomic nervous system arousal for which there is no top-down equivalent (Sharpe Lohrasbe & Ogden, 2017). Offering the somatic resources during EMDR Phase 2 can be a welcome addition to the usual EMDR suggestions for resourcing (non-somatic resources such as objects, services, relationships, attributes, etc.), which can also become somatic resources once steps are taken to embody them, again using SP techniques.

Another of the basic premises of EMDR and the AIP model is the use of free association in processing rather than narrowing the client's attention during Phase 4: Desensitization. Trusting AIP to guide where the client needs to focus, take in new information, and process relevant emotion works well with younger clients who are not so easily overwhelmed by the emotional and physiological. However, given the overwhelming nature of traumatic stress and the limited resources of those with less life experience and less than fully mature nervous systems, it may be wise and hold greater promise to limit the information a young person needs to process. Borrowing from the SP skills *framing* and *de-linking the building blocks of experience*, clients can manage the amount and intensity of traumatic reactions such that new information, the exploration of unsatisfying and problematic responses, and discovery of preferable responses can be processed.

Adaptations for Youth

Ricky Greenwald (1999) was one of the first to write about EMDR and adolescents' psychotherapy. He and others (Lovett, 1999; Tinker & Wilson, 1999) have provided practical suggestions for adapting the standard EMDR protocol for younger clients. There are several adaptations for youth which include adjusting for language capacities, explanation of concepts, use of age/stage relevant metaphors, incorporating greater degrees of imaginative solutions, drawing or other artwork, engaging the somatic narrative though physicalizing difficult dynamics, adding continuous bilateral stimulation to soothe or expedite processing depending on the phase (EMDR) or stage (SP) of the process.

EMDR's R-TEP protocol also holds similarities to SP's frame-by-frame processing of traumatic memory. Finally, some anecdotal success has been achieved through the addition of alternating bilateral stimulation (a feature of EMDR processing) to SP's sensorimotor sequencing.

Case Illustration

Kal

Kal was a 14-year-old who had been brought reluctantly to therapy by his single mother. Both Kal and his mother had become overwhelmed by his nightmares, anxiety, and what his mother feared was the beginnings of an eating disorder. The nightmares began when he was 5 or 6 and seemed to coincide with his parents contentious and ultimately abusive relationship ending in divorce. Before adolescence, his mother would allow him to sleep in her bed or she would be up several times in the night to soothe him from episodes of nightmares. The nightmares worsened after his mum insisted he sleep in his own bed.

The anxiety initially showed as nervousness around being away from his mother but over time seemed to increase, impacting Kal's friendships and participation in sports, and seemed also to relate to a constant habit of checking things – like house and car doors, backpacks, shoes, and the where-abouts of his mother at all hours of the day and night. Kal's eating concerns seemed to center around a growing suspicion that food was contaminated. When such fear was high, Kal would refuse to eat all but a sustenance diet.

In therapy, Kal had difficulty focusing as he recounted past and current events, the content of the nightmares, the thoughts and fear related to his "anxiety." We spent time helping Kal find somatic resources to mediate the hyperarousal of his nervous system. His preferred somatic resources were grounding, orienting, spinal alignment, and an embodied boundary. These were developed using a primarily SP approach which was enhanced occasionally with the use of bilateral taps to the backs of Kal's hands, or eye movements. Despite his ability to change state in session and often following nightmares, though it might take a few minutes, and also to reduce the frequency and intensity of his "anxiety" and eating symptoms, he still exceeded his window of tolerance during attempts to process traumatic experience.

We began to gain greater traction on his symptoms when SP concepts and techniques were included with the EMDR we were using. First, we used the concept *de-linking the building blocks of experience*. Kal was asked to attend to processing (desensitizing) that focused only on sensation and movement and excluded emotional and cognitive elements, for the first while. When a thought was expressed, Kal was gently directed to focus on the sensation or movement that went with the thought. With this he was able to process a great deal of his nightmares, and some of his recollections of his parents' fighting.

When he was able to tolerate noticing sensation or movement, we proceeded, and when it got too intense, we processed back to the window of tolerance, that is, to just notice the sensations until he felt back in his window and fully present. The final way we limited the amount and intensity of information was to use a reference point, a *frame*, rather than to go with free association. In this way we worked only with a moment in a nightmare or a memory (in SP it is often called a "sliver" of memory), such that we worked frame by frame through the memory as if it were a movie reel. This fit nicely with the EMDR metaphor of watching a movie or sitting on a train and watching the imagery flow by. Each frame's sensations were processed before proceeding to the next.

Over the course of a few months we had processed enough nightmares that they became a rare occurrence and were no longer fixated on past experiences. We worked through the major life stress of his parents' marriage and divorce, using fairly standard EMDR protocols, yet we maintained the bottom-up approach throughout the course of our work together. The other concerns around anxiety began to subside, as did the eating issues. Kal began to develop a friendship or two and, by the time he stopped therapy, he had joined an extracurricular school group.

Bibliography

Adler-Tapia, R. & Settle, C. (2017). *EMDR and the Art of Psychotherapy with Children: Infants to Adolescents*, 2nd ed. New York: Springer Publishing Company.

Bromberg, P.M. (2011). *The Shadow of the Tsunami: And the Growth of the Relational Mind*. New York: Routledge.

Gomez, A. (2013). *EMDR Therapy and Adjunct Approaches with Children: Complex Trauma, Attachment and Dissociation*. New York: Springer Publishing Company.

Greenwald, R. (1999). *Eye Movement Desensitization and Reprocessing (EMDR) in Child and Adolescent Psychotherapy*. Lanham, MD: Jason Aronson, Inc.

Lovett, J. (1999). *Small Wonders: Healing Childhood Trauma with EMDR*. New York: Free Press.

Ogden, P., Minton, K. & Pain, C. (2006). *Trauma and the Body: A Sensorimotor Approach to Psychotherapy*. New York: W.W. Norton.

Parnell, L. (2013). *Attachment Focused EMDR: Healing Relational Trauma*. New York: W. W. Norton.

Shapiro, F. (2001). *Eye Movement Reprocessing and Desensitization: Basic Principles, Protocols, and Procedures*, 2nd ed. New York: Guilford.

Sharpe Lohrasbe, R. (2015). Sensorimotor Considerations in EMDR: Preparation and Processing. Presentation at the EMDR Canada Annual Conference, Vancouver, BC.

Sharpe Lohrasbe, R. & Ogden, P. (2017). Somatic Resources: Sensorimotor Psychotherapy Approach to Stabilizing Arousal in Child and Family Treatment. *Australia and New Zealand Journal of Child and Family Therapy*, 38(4): 573–581.

Soloman, R. & Shapiro, F. (2008). EMDR and the Adaptive Information Processing Model: Potential Mechanisms of Change. *Journal of EMDR Practice and Research*, 2(4): 315–325.

Tinker, R. & Wilson, S. (1999). *Through the Eyes of a Child: EMDR with Children*. New York: W. W. Norton.

van der Kolk, B. (2001). Foreword. In Shapiro, F.. *Eye Movement Reprocessing and Desensitization: Basic Principles, Protocols, and Procedures*, 2nd ed. New York: Guilford.

Wesselmann, D., Schweitzer, C. & Armstrong, S. (2014). *Integrative Team Treatment for Attachment Trauma in Children: Family Therapy and EMDR*. New York: W. W. Norton.

Part II

Essential Components in Clinical Work with Complexly Traumatized Youth

3 Comprehensive Trauma Assessment

A comprehensive assessment is critical prior to beginning treatment. Assessment, however, spans the duration of therapy. It has been my experience, far too often, that the unasked questions reveal the underlying issues that become the focus of clinical attention. For example, caregivers may seek services at a children's mental health agency for their child due to behavior issues at home, in school, in social settings, or sometimes across multiple domains. A comprehensive assessment allows the clinician to identify patterns of family interaction that might factor in to the presenting problems, to pinpoint areas that are particularly challenging, and to uncover previous life experiences, such as surgery or loss, or an unrecognized trauma, that contribute to the presenting concerns. Additionally, the assessment identifies strengths and resources to utilize in client engagement and to build competence and mastery over the course of treatment. Whenever possible, the assessment is completed with youth and caregivers. I inform all persons present that they may opt to say "defer" if they choose not to share information with others present, and that we will meet later in various configurations, as appropriate. With adolescents, I prefer to complete some of the items, such as the time line, early in the assessment to give them a sense of control in the process and an opportunity to feel connected (i.e. establish rapport). Other variables to consider during the assessment and treatment processes, such as prosody and proximity, are detailed in later chapters.

For reference purposes, an assessment template is provided at the end of this chapter. Following is a detailed description about each section of the assessment template. Note that this template is the culmination of 25 years of experience working at various agencies, in front-line and supervisory/training capacities, in the US and Canada, and it contains information that I consider useful for the trauma assessment process. Alternating pronouns (e.g. she/he/they) appear throughout the text. The order and contents have been refined over the years as I have used it for consultation and teaching purposes, and as I have expanded my own knowledge and experience. For example, recent research, including dissemination of the ACEs study, has identified impairment in self-regulation as a serious consequence of complex trauma, and so questions specific to regulation were added to this template about five years ago. Consider the template a guide. Over time, clinicians tend to automate the process based on their own styles and clinical work settings, and are able to collect necessary information without the use of a template or form. With experience, this process becomes a clinical interview rather than a structured process.

Prior to beginning the assessment process, the potential risks and benefits of assessment and treatment must be covered. Informed consent includes knowing what potential challenges may arise along the way. For example, I often let caregivers know that there may be an increase in symptoms or behaviors during the early stages of treatment while their child unpacks or works through issues they had previously ignored or were unaware of. Additionally, the limits of confidentiality must be addressed with caregivers and the youth. As mandated reporters, we must be clear with them that disclosure that suggests past or present harm to a child must be reported. Various creative tools are useful when reviewing family dynamics (e.g. genogram), historical information (e.g. a time line), and the youth's ability to recognize, manage, and express emotions (Body Feelings Map – BFM). Samples and descriptions of these tools are given at the end of the chapter, with the exception of the BFM which is detailed in Chapter 8, and forms are included in the appendices.

Risks, Benefits, and Limits of Confidentiality

Risks of assessment and treatment may include the following:

* increased symptomology (e.g. more intense or frequent nightmares);
* new concerning behaviors (e.g. the child is attending school again but she is isolating herself in her bedroom most evenings);
* increased conflict in family relationships at home as members adjust to the safety and willingness to share thoughts and feelings in sessions;
* the revelation of issues that caregivers had previously been unaware of.

Advise caregivers and the youth that assessment and treatment can be triggering and ensure them that we will monitor and intervene as necessary (e.g. if the youth's self-injurious behavior or eating disorder worsens). Safety planning is sometimes done at the assessment phase when suicidal thoughts are endorsed.

Benefits may include:

* reduction or resolution of concerns;
* improved social or family (interpersonal) relationships;
* a general positive "ripple affect" across domains (e.g. the youth's presenting concerns revolved around academics and as she works through this issue, we may observe improvements in social functioning as well);
* the youth is returned to the appropriate place on his developmental trajectory (e.g. by working through his historical abuse, he will learn about age-appropriate and healthy sexuality, thereby increasing his ability to have intimate relationships as an adult).

Confidentiality

A standard description of confidentiality (e.g. what is said in here stays in here) is augmented with limitations including:

- if something shared leads to suspicion that a minor is at risk of harm (or has been harmed);
- if there is a statement describing an intention to kill someone;
- for minor youth, suicidal plans are shared with caregivers who are responsible for their safety;
- if a form authorizing exchange of information between past or present service providers has been signed;
- if the file is subpoenaed by court.

A quick note about treatment planning before we dive into the assessment template: the process of treatment planning is not covered in this book but does play a role in treatment. Effective treatment plans are assessment-informed and include opportunities to augment strengths and reduce areas of concern (Ford et al., 2013). Agencies tend to use very structured treatment plans with clear goals. For example, an agency might use the acronym SMART (specific, measurable, achievable, realistic, time-bound). Treatment plans can be seen as healing maps; they enable transparency and encourage collaboration between service providers and clients. Some settings assess progress and reevaluate every three to six months.

Assessment Template – Section Descriptions and Suggestions

Section A: Basic Demographic and Systems Information

The initial section captures basic client, family, and academic information. Data here includes the youth's full name and date of birth, pronoun preferences, name(s) of caregiver(s), referral source, involvement of child protection services, custody and access or adoption details, and information about the client's current living situation. The living situation lists others who reside with the youth. The latter point is important as we may have to refer to these details, should we require the involvement of children's protection services. We also want to inquire about cultural, traditional, or religious beliefs or customs to consider in treatment. Additionally, academic information, such as school, grade, and academic performance, is collected. Ask about special education and whether there is an IEP (Individual Educational Plan) for the youth. Finally, ask the youth and caregiver what they see as the presenting problem or the concerns that brought them to your office today. I typically ask the youth first as this is experienced as empowering in a situation where they often feel they do not have any say. Also, it is good to have a sense of whether they have been informed of the reasons for the visit. Youth, especially younger children, may simply repeat what a caregiver says so it is recommended that youth be given an opportunity to share their own thoughts. Know that younger children may not be able to articulate themselves here, as well as throughout the assessment process, so offer them drawing or play materials to assist with communication.

Section B: Past and Present Providers, Developmental and Medical History

We obtain a list of past and present service providers as we may want to connect with them now or later in treatment. If we think we might want to share information, remember that we must have written consent to share. It is important to share information with present providers since you want to be working toward the same goals rather than at cross-purposes. As noted earlier in Adele's vignette, her other provider and I disagreed on a course of action for self-injurious behaviors. We want to clear up any confusion for the child and/or caregiver and we also want to ensure that we adhere to ethical responsibilities. At some point you may want to coordinate with prescribing psychiatrists or school counsellors; thus it is best to know who else is involved before treatment commences. Additionally, this will provide us with a sense of the ways the caregiver has sought (or not) assistance in the past. For example, have they worked with various providers for the same issue(s)? If so, what precipitated the changes in provider? Chapter 6 provides a discussion of diagnostic dilemmas that may be useful when considering information shared by other service providers.

In this section, we also document past and current medications. Documentation of medication is important as it reflects caregivers' attempts at providing effective medication, and we want a record of any side effects the child experienced with medications. You also want to obtain details for any other allergies. For example, clients might be allergic to lavender or peanuts so you want to ensure these items are not present during their sessions.

Developmental history is about milestones (walking, talking, toilet training), birth and pregnancy (e.g. was it a healthy pregnancy? was it planned? any issues with delivery, did the mother experience post-partum depression?), and skill acquisition (e.g. was his speech delayed? did the child see a speech and language therapist?). We also want to ask about fine and gross motor skills in earlier years, as well as social skills. For example, did the child have difficulty making or maintaining friendships when younger? If so, what changed these difficulties? If working with younger children, we might inquire about day care, especially in relation to social-emotional development. Finally, inquire about any other developmental concerns that the caregiver might have.

Section C: Family Background and History

It is helpful to begin this section with a genogram. Genogram symbols are provided at the end of this chapter. The genogram is not only an engaging, creative way to gather information about family patterns and dynamics, current and intergenerational, but it also gives the child an opportunity to view and discuss their trauma in a larger, external context (Wieland, 1998). This can be healing for a child who has blamed herself for what has happened to her.

Other areas to explore here include discipline or parenting style, extended family involvement and relationships, sibling relationships, family history of mental illness and substance use/abuse, medical conditions, and legal system involvement. Again, all of this information will be captured and coded with color on the genogram for a single-page snapshot of the family history and patterns. Ask about the number and frequency of moves, and reasons for moving, to be covered on the time line later as well. Frequent moves may underlie challenges the child faced such as difficulty with social skills and academic setbacks.

Section D: Trauma/Abuse History, Substance Use

Depending on the youth's age, they may decide to defer substance use information for a later time when the caregiver is not present. Some youth may also deny past/present use but may share with us later when they are completing the time line. Sometimes this section offers an opportunity for psychoeducation about what constitutes various forms of abuse. As with earlier sections, the genogram may capture abuse and trauma history for the youth and we can carry that information forward here.

Section E: Mental Status Exam (MSE)

The Mental Status Exam is a carry-over from my graduate school training. As far as I know, most clinicians do not evaluate these areas in an assessment. I like to document this information as baseline data and some of the features, such as affect or motor activity, will be tracked over the course of treatment. Should you decide to use this section, consider that the responses circled are subjective as they are your observations, and the youth's mood (e.g. might be anxious or angry about being there) can impact their initial presentation. Most of the MSE is self-explanatory; however, elaboration on a couple of items follows.

Perceptual Disturbance

Ask the youth if they ever see or hear things that are not there. Ask about voices that tell or ask them to do things. For younger children, like toddlers, an imaginary best friend is normal developmentally. However, children typically outgrow magical thinking around 10 years of age and it is a red flag, requiring further exploration, if an older child is exhibiting magical thinking. Waters (2016) discusses the importance of exploring warning signs of dissociation in children. The topic of dissociation is covered later in Chapter 12.

Orientation

Simple questions to assess their orientation to person, place, and time include:

> What is your full name and how old are you?
> What city do you live in?
> What season is this? Or, what day of the week is this?

Section F: Concerns

This section is a checklist of areas that might contribute to the presenting concerns. By this point, the caregiver or youth may have already endorsed some items so this will offer opportunity for elaboration. Indicate whether the concern is past or present, and seek details about frequency, impact, and when the concern first appeared. If the concerns existed in the past, inquire about start and end times.

Section G: Skills/Abilities, Resources (Individual and Family)

We want to ask about skills and resources that can be enhanced. Questions in this section enlighten the youth and caregiver about resources they may not have considered and can foster a sense of hope. Gather information about the youth's capacity to regulate. We might ask the caregiver, "Tell me about how X expresses their feelings," or "What does X do when she is angry…sad, etc.?" For conflict management, ask about what the youth does when she disagrees with someone. With the self-soothing question, for example, inquire about the ways the youth calms himself down or is able to manage sadness or disappointment. We will gain information about the family's patterns of emotional expression as well. For example, which feelings are acceptable/unacceptable? Does the family freely express a range of emotions, or is there a tendency to push feelings inside? Are there consequences (e.g. minimizing, dismissing, embarrassing) for open expression? Note that we are observing nonverbal communication of caregivers and youth throughout the assessment process and this may be a particularly illuminating section for observations. Verbalized content and nonverbal expression may be incongruent. For example, the caregiver might say, "He's never angry, nobody in our house ever gets angry," but her jaw and throat are tensed and her son shoots a glance at her with his raised eyebrows. Lastly, explore the youth's awareness of personal space and boundaries. Often, more information about family dynamics and boundaries is shared here. Make note of concerns that may require psychoeducation or clinical attention later.

Section H: Strengths (Individual and Family)

Obtain a description, in verbatim as much as possible, of the child's perception of his own strengths. This can be done with art or play activities, if necessary, with younger children. Then, invite the caregivers to share what they consider the child's individual strengths, and what they consider family strengths. Inquire about protective factors, such as systemic, familial, or extra-familial aspects that are viewed as contributing to the overall well-being of the youth and family. We may have gleaned protective factors from information previously collected. Next, gather a list of interests from the youth. These can be utilized later in treatment, both as a way to engage the youth and to keep therapy interesting for them. Additionally, I like to ask the youth what they would wish for if they could be granted three wishes. Some clever children will respond, "More wishes." I like to ask the question at the end of this part of the assessment because it offers an opportunity for the youth to be playful and use their imagination; furthermore, unmet needs could possibly be uncovered. Finally, I ask the child and caregiver what would be different three months from now if treatment were beneficial for them. Depending on the age of the child and their understanding of therapy, I might use something like "our meetings together" instead of "treatment."

Section I: Summary of Needs (Individual and Family); Recommendations for Further Assessment

The remainder of the assessment form is completed after meeting with the youth and family. These questions inform treatment planning and further assessment. You may have already decided that psychometrics would be beneficial (e.g. it is clear to you that there are trauma symptoms and you want to back up your clinical interview), and that consents to share information are required.

Psychometric Descriptions

Note: There are limitations on the use of measures depending on the regulatory or licensing body. For example, those registered with a College of Psychologists can administer and score all tools listed; however, other professions, such as social workers or psychotherapists, may be able to administer some but not all. Refer to the test purchasing instructions for permissions. Also note that many of these measures are intended to screen rather than diagnose.

Measure	Age Range	Domains Assessed	Format, Features, Author
A-DES (Adolescent Dissociative Experiences Scale)	11–18 years	Dissociation	Screening tool Self-report 30 items Armstrong et al.
CBCL (Child Behaviour Checklist)	6–18 years (also a version for younger children ages 1.5–5)	Anxiety/mood / somatic (internalizing), Behavior concerns (externalizing)	Caregiver, teacher reports (TRF), self-report (YSR) T. Achenbach

(continued)

(Cont.)

Measure	Age Range	Domains Assessed	Format, Features, Author
CDC (Child Dissociative Checklist)	Not indicated	Dissociation	Screening tool Caregiver report 20 items F. Putnam et al.
CDI 2 (Children's Depression Inventory)	7–17 years	Negative mood, Ineffectiveness, Negative self-esteem, anhedonia, interpersonal problems	Self-report Caregiver, teacher reports 27 items M. Kovacs
CSBI (Children's Sexual Behavior Inventory)	2–12 years	Measures sexual behavior in children in 9 areas	Caregiver report 38 items W. Friedrich
MASC-2 (Multidimensional Anxiety Scale for Children)	8–19 years	Anxiety	Self-report Caregiver report J. March
TSCC (Trauma Symptom Checklist for Children)	8–16 years	Anger, anxiety, depression, PTSD, somatic concerns, dissociation, sexual concerns	Self-report 54 items Briere, et al. (1996)
TSCYC (Trauma Symptom Checklist for Young Children)	3–12 years	Anxiety/mood, traumatic stress symptoms, sexual concerns	Caregiver report 90 items Briere et al.
UCLA-PTSD	6 years and younger, child/ adolescent	DSM-5 PTSD criteria	Youth, caregiver Steinberg et al. – updated for DSM-5 Training video available
YCPC (Young Child PTSD Checklist)	1–6 years	Trauma history/ exposure, PTSD symptoms	Caregiver report M. Schreeninga

Basic Genogram Symbols

There is a range among professionals regarding genogram symbols. For simplicity, the basic symbols are provided here.

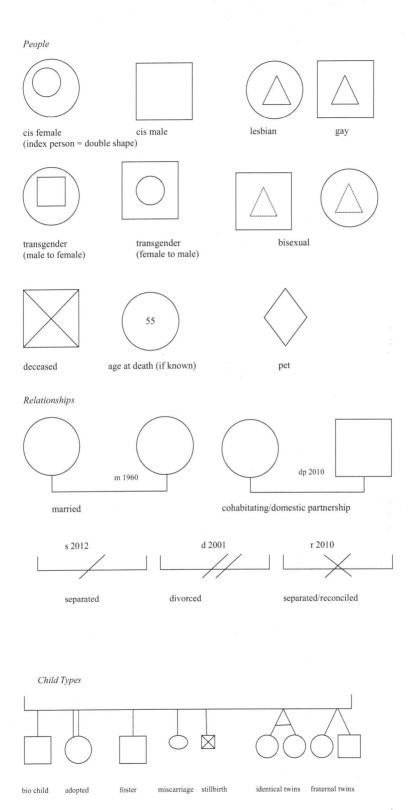

People

cis female
(index person = double shape)

cis male

lesbian

gay

transgender
(male to female)

transgender
(female to male)

bisexual

deceased

55

age at death (if known)

pet

Relationships

m 1960

married

dp 2010

cohabitating/domestic partnership

s 2012

separated

d 2001

divorced

r 2010

separated/reconciled

Child Types

bio child   adopted   foster   miscarriage   stillbirth   identical twins   fraternal twins

Relationship Dynamics

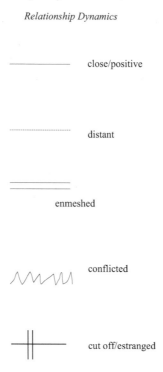

——————————   close/positive

·······················   distant

══════════   enmeshed

close/positive

distant

enmeshed

conflicted

cut off/estranged

Patterns/Intergenerational Transmission

Once all family members (immediate and extended over two generations) are included, ask about the following areas:

Mental health: green dot – list suspected/diagnosed

Substance use: orange dot – list substance and whether active/past use (include misuse or overuse of prescription drugs, pot, crack, etc.)

Other addictions: yellow dot – list and indicate whether current/past (include internet, porn, shopping, gambling, etc.)

Domestic violence: brown lines with directional arrows between persons (partners or caregiver/child); list types – P (physical), V (verbal), E (emotional), F (financial), Ps (Psychological)

Legal issues: purple dot – list

Sexual abuse: red lines with directional arrows – list age/duration of the abuse

Physical/medical: blue dot – list condition such as cancer, diabetes, heart issues, etc.

Include other factors such as suicide, homicide as appropriate.

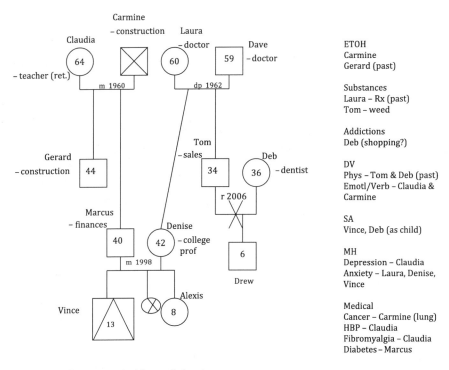

Figure 3.1 Genogram (without Colors)

Time Line

The Time Line activity is part of the assessment. It captures the youth's significant events and may present themes (e.g. loss, injury, lack of control, hopeless world view, etc.) in the youth's life. Also, it is a relatively innocuous exercise that facilitates therapeutic rapport and identifies areas of concern (e.g. memory/time confusion, cognitive limitations) early in treatment. The Time Line activity is presented to the youth as part of all assessment processes and they are assured that there is no right or wrong way to complete it. I like to begin by inviting them to select a sheet of paper that is their favorite color (favorite color is filed away in my mind for later reference) and then I introduce the activity something like this:

> Today we are going to work on a Time Line activity. I invite all new kids to complete this because it gives us a great picture of all the things you have experienced in your life over time. We will begin by choosing a sheet of paper that's your favorite color (ask youth to select from a stack of colored paper that includes white, should they not want a colored sheet or report that they have no favorite color). Ok, now what year were you born again?

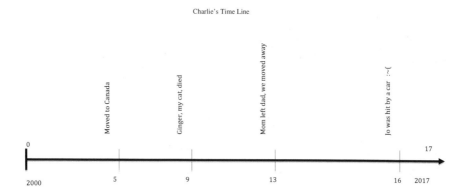

Figure 3.2 Time Line

Right, and this is (current year) so you are how old again? *Note: Some kids will laugh or be annoyed that you have forgotten their age or year of birth, so I just roll with it and let them know that numbers and math are not my forte. You are essentially modeling that it is okay to be imperfect.*

Next, I draw a line on the bottom of a sheet (see Figure 3.2 above) with birth year at one end and current year/child's age at the other side of the page. I comment on the arrowhead drawn on the right side (current year) being right here, right now, thus planting the seeds for mindfulness. The client is then given the page and asked to think about three to five memories or events that stand out in his memory. Clients often ask if it has to be good or bad things, and they are assured that any memory or event can go on the time line if it is important to them. Sometimes I suggest they imagine their life is a movie, like those old-fashioned film reels, and if we were to freeze frame on the most important or memorable events, that is what we want to include. I ask them to put little hatch marks, like I did for the birth and current years, and then add a few words for each event. They are assured we will talk about each event once all have been added.

Once all the events have been included, we discuss each to gain an understanding of the relevance, and I ask them to share how they feel now when they talk about the particular events. If we plan to use EMDR in the future, I will also get a SUD (subjective unit of distress) at this time. As necessary, details are jotted onto the time line. With the example in Figure 3.2, Charlie's memories seem to have a theme of loss, for example. At this point I would not reflect that for the client, but make a mental note again. The next step is flipping the page over, drawing a line that is a continuation of the other side, and ending with question marks as we cannot know what year goes at the end. This side is labeled (client's) Future. It is not unusual for traumatized youth to struggle with this task. Many are experiencing a sense of hopelessness and foreshortened future. Ask the youth to write down three to five goals or plans for their future, along with the age or age range they expect to reach the goal. If they have difficulty coming up with something, I might throw out general suggestions such as: "Is there a place you want to travel one day?"; "What do you want to do after high school?"; "Is there a kind of pet you've always wanted?" This activity can be diagnostic in the client's ability to see past their present.

Trauma Assessment – Child/Adolescent

SECTION A

Child's Name	
DOB	
Caregiver/Guardian(s)	
Referral Source	
CAS Involvement?	
Custody/Adoption?	
Current Living Situation/ Family Constellation	
Cultural/Religious	
School/Grade	
IEP/Special Ed?	
Other Providers?	

Child's Perception of Presenting Situation
Caregiver Perception

SECTION B

Previous Services/Service Providers			
Date(s)	Agency/Person	Type of Service	Details

Other Current Providers (e.g. Pediatrician, Psychiatrist)

Current/Past Medication(s)?
Current
Previous

Allergy Information

Medical/Surgical/Hospitalization History

Developmental History	
Pregnancy/Birth	
Milestones	
Language	

Developmental History	
Cognitive	
Academic	
Motor/Coordination	
Social	
Other	

SECTION C

Family History – complete and attach genogram	
Caregiver/Guardian Relationship History	
Communication Style	
Discipline Style	
Moves (freq./reason)	
Extended Family Relationships	
Sibling Relationships	
Substance Abuse	
Mental Illness	
Medical Conditions	
Legal Involvement	
Other	

SECTION D

Abuse/Trauma History – circle and provide details	
None physical neglect verbal emotional domestic violence exposure sexual abuse	
Victim of	
Victim of	
Engaged in Acts of	
Significant Separation/Loss	

Substance Use/Addictions – list substance, age of first and last use, frequency, any adverse effects (include cigarettes, alcohol, weed, internet, gambling, sex, etc.)	

SECTION E

MSE
Interaction
friendly   cooperative   hostile/angry   anxious   evasive   detached guarded   bored   other_____
Motor activity
Normal   hyperactive listless   fidgety   slowed   facial tics body tics   other_____
Affect
Full range/approp. to content   incongruent   flat   labile   intense/reactive Other_____
Perceptual disturbance
No evidence of psychosis   hallucinations (audio/visual)   delusional/magical thinking Other_____
Orientation
Person   place   time   situation
Appearance
Neat/clean   unkempt   heavy   thin   average weight   poor hygiene other
Speech

SECTION F

	Areas of Concern – circle past or present and provide details		
past present	Aggression/violence toward others	past present	Self-injury
past present	Property destruction	past present	Suicidal thoughts/talk/ attempts
past present	Anxious/panic attacks	past present	Eating disorder/binging/ purging/picky
past present	Sleep disturbance/ nightmares	past present	Depressed mood/ sadness
past present	Hallucinations/delusions/ paranoia	past present	Fire-setting or cruelty to animals
past present	Social withdrawal/isolation	past present	Rapid mood changes
past present	Homicidal thoughts/ behavior	past present	Sexual concerns
past present	Truancy/academic concerns	past present	Impulsive/inattentive/ distractible
past present	Running away	past present	Legal issues
past present	Stealing/vandalism	past present	Obsessive/compulsive behavior
past present	Needs to be in control	past present	Enuresis/Encopresis
past present	Body image	past present	Aversion to touch/ sensory issues
past present	Self-concept	past present	Other

SECTION G

Skills/Abilities – check and provide details as relevant		
Personal hygiene		Family resources
Household chores		Coping skills/emotional management
Nutrition		Leisure/recreation
Personal safety		
Other		

Resources – check and provide details as relevant		
Housing		Healthcare
Transportation		Family/social
Educational		Community involvement/support
Financial		Other

Regulation
Able to tolerate and express strong emotions such as anger, frustration, sadness. Please provide details.
Able to tolerate and manage conflict. Please provide details.
Able to self-soothe. Please provide details.
Able to form and maintain healthy relationships, and demonstrates awareness of age-appropriate boundaries. Please provide details.

SECTION H

Strengths
Individual/family strengths (per child):
Individual/family strengths (per caregiver):
Protective factors:
Interests:
Three wishes:

SECTION I

Summary of needs – check all that apply:
- risk of harm to self
- risk of harm to others
- inability to demonstrate age-appropriate daily living skills
- inability to function in a school setting
- need for assistance from multiple community services
- needs cannot be met on an outpatient basis

Recommended for further assessment:
- TSCC/TSCYC (or similar trauma measure)
- MASC (or similar anxiety measure)
- CDI (or similar depression measure)
- Other
- Attachments
- Consents signed

Assessment completed by (name, credentials)_____,_____on _____.

Signature of assessor_____.

4   Guiding Treatment Principles

As we begin this section, let us reflect on the Latin adage *Primun non nocere* (first, do no harm).

How can we strive toward this as a minimal goal? Sometimes doing no harm entails doing nothing. Sounds peculiar, right? Consider empowering a youth who has to return to a violent home situation: what we see as growth-enhancing could increase his risk of harm at home. Guiding principles are a series of premises that we can use to guide our work with traumatized children and families. The principles are interconnected and touch upon all of our work. Many clinical authors include a list of guiding treatment principles in their material (e.g. Boon, Steele & van der Hart, 2011: James, 1989; Saxe, Ellis & Kaplow, 2007; Waters, 2016).

Working with traumatized children and youth requires an understanding of theory, such as attachment and child development, knowledge about current legislation surrounding child protection and mandated reporting requirements, and the willingness to keep abreast of emergent best practices. But working with youth also requires skills and qualities that are less tangible than theory and legislation. Anyone who has done trauma work knows how quickly we can move through a range of emotions with our clients, from anger to sadness to fear and joy, but there is another feeling we experience in this important work: hope. We have hope as we join them on their healing journeys that we can facilitate the return to their developmental trajectories, and we hope that we can provide a supportive environment that nourishes their potential for happy, safe, connected adult lives. These principles are based on experiences within agencies and private practice; thus, I appreciate that there may be limitations and restrictions to adherence. It is my hope that agencies include these principles in their clinicians' orientations and their interagency policy and procedure manuals.

Let us begin with whom to include in the treatment process. Best practice calls for the involvement of caregivers but that is not always possible. Not only is it helpful to have supportive, trusted caregivers on board throughout the course of treatment but also, especially with younger children, caregivers play a crucial role in co-regulating (expanded upon in Chapter 7), monitoring, and facilitating enhancement of coping techniques in the home. If the youth's caregivers do not share a home, ensure that consent for treatment has been obtained from all parties involved in the youth's caretaking decisions. Sometimes this requires separate meetings with the adults. Individual meetings with caregivers are also important because there is often information caregivers have to share that might not be appropriate for the youth to be privy to; moreover, we want to increase the likelihood of having caregivers on board to ensure treatment completion. Other collaterals to include, particularly during completion of the comprehensive assessment, are educators, child protective services and legal authorities (if involved), and, possibly, extended family. Note that the principles are not listed in any particular order and we often attend to several simultaneously.

1. Safe Setting or Environment

The first impression is crucial. Is the office space inviting? Does it offer visual stimulation that is interesting yet not overwhelming? Is the décor age-appropriate? Depending on whom we are seeing for the session, we may want to rearrange furniture. For example, if we know a family is attending an intake meeting, we want to ensure there is adequate seating available. Research has shown that sound or noise plays a role in sensing safety. In his writing on the Polyvagal Theory, Porges (2017) posits that we should strive to eliminate or reduce low frequency sounds. His theory proposes that threat is neurocepted with the presence of low frequency sounds; thus, it may be difficult for a young person, already on the edges of or outside their window of tolerance, to feel safe in such a setting. Similarly, our prosody can either foster a sense of safety or send the youth further outside their window of tolerance.

How we speak and engage with the youth plays a role in feeling safe. Ogden (2013) notes: "Most obvious and transparent is the explicit exchange of words, but the implicit conversation that goes on beneath the words is argu-ably more important." (p. 35). Wieland (2017) espouses the need to consider the caregiver's feelings of safety as well. Thus, it is essential that we be mindful of our gestures, facial expressions, and body language in initial and ongoing interactions with youth and their caregivers. Included here is the importance of "fit." The pivotal role the therapeutic relationship plays in therapy effectiveness is well documented, with estimates suggesting 70% of therapy effectiveness is based on the client–therapist relationship. Waters (2016) notes: "Having a positive relationship with the child is a prerequisite for providing the structure for trauma processing." (p. 288). We must also be mindful of having a good fit with the caregivers. The compassion we feel and offer our young clients must be extended to caregivers. Caregivers often present as frustrated and overwhelmed by the challenges they are dealing with and we need to offer val-idation and support for their experiences. When possible, offer complimentary consultation meetings so that the clients have an opportunity to sense whether there is a good fit. We also have to be mindful of the challenge when we work with youth and caregivers or other family members: we might be a good fit with the youth but not the caregiver. Lack of fit can result in attrition.

2. Safety and Stabilization First (Phase One)

Safety and stabilization are our first priority. Regardless of the approach or model we use, experts agree that we must attend to this prior to working through the trauma (Fisher, 1999; Herman, 1992; Ogden, 2006; Rothschild, 2017; Wieland, 1998). We want to ensure the child has a supportive, nurturing home setting. If we suspect they do not, we must remember our requirements to report suspected abuse/neglect/exposure to DV, for example. It is unsettling that we may jeopardize ongoing work with youth once we make a call to child protection services. When possible, I inform the caregiver that a call must be made and attempt to include them in the process. Of course, this is not always possible and we risk losing the client. As noted earlier, caregivers may lack the capacity to regulate themselves and thus cannot co-regulate their child, necessitating work focusing on the caregiver's sense of safety at the onset of treatment.

Exploring and enhancing resources is part of phase one in trauma treatment. During the assessment, we inquire about existing resources (Ogden & Fisher, 2015). For example, do walks in nature alleviate her suicidal thoughts? Does he play guitar to elevate his mood and energy levels? Do they find a quiet corner and listen to soothing music when feeling overwhelmed or stressed? All clients have resources; we just need to ask the right questions to elicit them and then expand on them.

3. Comprehensive Assessment

It is preferable that the same clinician completes the assessment and provides treatment. Some agencies offer separate programs for assessment and treatment, so this is not always feasible. Using the same clinician benefits the client in many ways, such as facilitating rapport from the start, and eliminating the need for the client to repeat the story. During the assessment, clinicians need to gather as much information as possible. Information gathering means asking a lot of questions, including the difficult questions. If we avoid going into the tough stuff, we risk indirectly messaging that we cannot handle the tough stuff. In TF-CBT, this is considered part of establishing baseline data and the beginning of the gradual in vivo desensitization process (Cohen et al., 2006). This must be done, however, while considering the child's window of tolerance and their capacity to self-regulate. Following is an illustration of a child outside her window of tolerance during the assessment. I was observing the assessment and intervened when the assessor did not stop the assessment despite the girl's obvious signs of distress.

> Kay was a 12-year old girl referred to a children's mental health center. Based on the "presenting problems" and her history it was determined that she was a suitable candidate for the TF-CBT research project. A lead agency conducted the assessment with the understanding that the client would receive treatment from another (my) agency. From the outset, Kay presented as cooperative and engaged. I observed that her leg shook constantly, her voice softened and her

eye contact decreased over the course of the first few hours. Her caregiver, interviewed separately, presented as unsupportive and, at times, hostile. We later learned that Kay's mother did not believe the abuse occurred and she resented being mandated to treatment by child protection services.

As the assessment proceeded into details about the sexual abuse (gathering baseline data), Kay appeared increasingly distressed: responses to questions were shorter, her voice was soft and tremulous, breathing appeared nonexistent, and eye contact diminished. Nonetheless, the assessor continued eliciting details about a particular incident of abuse. Kay's dysregulation peaked and the juice she was drinking exploded through her nose and mouth. She expressed an apology and began rocking back and forth in her seat. At this point I interrupted the assessment and suggested that we go for a walk. Kay and I went to the gym to shoot some hoops. During this activity, I offered reassuring words, expressed empathy for Kay's experience, and used basketball to co-regulate Kay (rhythm, movement, an attuned supportive other). When she no longer appeared distressed, as evidenced by a decrease in the symptoms listed above, we returned to the assessment room. Having been restored to a place of homeostasis, and gained a sense of safety in relationship to someone whom she believed she could trust, Kay was able to continue the assessment process.

4. Trauma-Focused versus Trauma-Informed Treatment

Much has been written about the importance of creating trauma-informed systems. Most agencies and organizations offer trauma-informed care (TIC) or trauma-informed practice (TIP). Trauma-informed care strives to recognize and understand all forms of trauma (e.g. physical, psychological) and the impact on the individual's (and their family's) life (Clark et al., 2015; Haskell, 2003). There is a focus on safety for clients (e.g. physical, psychological) and service providers. Numerous trauma-informed practice guides are available for those who wish to learn more about TIC/TIP (e.g. http://bccewh.bc.ca/wp-content/uploads/2012/05/2013_TIP-Guide.pdf; http://trauma-informed.ca/wp-content/uploads/2013/10/Trauma-informed_Toolkit.pdf). Trauma-informed care is an overall approach that focuses on safety and strengths rather than pathologizing the individual.

While TIC considers knowledge about trauma and strives to include this in all aspects of service delivery (e.g. assessment, treatment, case management), it may not address specific trauma-related symptoms. This is where trauma-focused treatment comes in. A recent example involved an 8-year-old girl referred to me by a trauma-informed occupational therapy agency. The agency employed sensory integration and principles of the SMART model (see Chapter 2), and they recognized that the girl required trauma-focused treatment: she disclosed sexual abuse and there was a flood of dysregulation that followed. The OT recognized the limitations of their scope of practice (see principle 14) and made a referral.

Trauma-focused treatment utilizes evidence-based and best practice treatment models that have been proven to facilitate recovery from trauma. There is a growing body of research (e.g. Cloitre, 2015) advocating for clinicians to look beyond the structured limitations of trauma-focused treatments as they tend to be cognitive-based (e.g. TF-CBT) and overlook the needs of complex trauma survivors. (See also: Evidence-Based Treatment for Adult Women with Child Abuse-Related Complex PTSD: A Quantitative Review, October 2014, *European Journal of Psychotraumatology*.) On the pro side, trauma-focused treatments directly address the impact of trauma on an individual's life and facilitate healing. All trauma-specific treatment models should be individualized to meet a particular client's needs, and consider the role of the therapeutic alliance in client safety.

5. Culturally Responsive, Anti-oppressive Framework

Treatment interventions are most effective when they consider the client's culture (Osofsky, 2011; Rubens et al., 2018). By culture here, I am referring to a broad range of factors such as ethnicity, religion, customs and beliefs, systemic oppression (e.g. heterosexism, misogyny, cultural oppression), and socioeconomic status. Furthermore, we need to be aware of our own cultural biases and background (Wieland, 2017). If we are unfamiliar or unsure, we can be curious with our clients, in a respectful, nonintrusive way, or we can do our own research to better prepare us to do the work with a child and family. We also need to be aware of systemic factors that impact our client and family, such as the historical treatment of Indigenous people in Canada. It is shocking and heartbreaking to know that the legacy continues to impact the Indigenous communities: nearly 50% of incarcerated youth in Canada are Indigenous (Stats Can 2016). Research on epigenetics and intergenerational transmission of trauma with Indigenous people and Holocaust survivors has identified mental health concerns in the current generation, including higher rates of depression and predisposition to PTSD following stressors (Bombay, Matheson & Anisman, 2013; Walters et al., 2011; Yehuda & Bierer, 2009).

While having dinner with a friend one evening, we were talking about intergenerational transmission of trauma and epigenetics in relation to Indigenous people and the Holocaust. My friend shared that she was a product of Canada's infamous "sixties scoop." Susan, my friend, agreed to share some of her story, particularly what mattered to her as an Indigenous child taken from her home and family. Following are her thoughts about the experience:

> I don't know how old I was when we were taken and put into foster homes. The foster homes were horrible, but when I was about 6 a white, missionary family adopted us. They were a good family, and they adopted both of us (Susan and her younger brother). We were not made to feel ashamed of our heritage and, since we lived near a reservation and my father was a missionary there, we were able to stay connected to our traditions and culture. I wish I still spoke my language (Cree) and had spent more time with

the elders to hear about the traditions, but I think overall I was lucky that I did not end up in a family that tried to change who I was.

With Indigenous children, maintaining connection to cultural identity is important to the healing process. A Government of Canada program, Aboriginal Head Start in Urban and Northern Communities (AHSUNC), of 2013 suggests the following to help foster a child's identity:

- Learn as much as you can about the child's culture – traditions, strengths, challenges.
- Balance the physical, emotional, mental, and spiritual dimensions.
- Support the child to learn/maintain traditional language.
- Seek and provide opportunities to engage in traditional activities, and to participate in community events (e.g. ceremonial events).
- Encourage interaction with community elders, to learn from their wisdom.
- Provide the child with books and videos (or links to videos) of traditional dance, games, and music.
- Speak openly about discrimination and systemic oppression, and microaggressions.

Following are some examples of using a culturally responsive, anti-oppressive framework:

One of my first jobs working with children and youth was at a children's mental health center in Atlanta, Georgia. I lived in Georgia for five years and experienced a very different culture than my native home, Toronto, Canada. Religion played a big role in most of my southern clients' lives. I found ways to use this as a resource in their treatment, such as increasing social interaction through church youth groups. However, I also witnessed the use of religion to justify harming a child. For example, one young client lived in a foster home. His foster mother repeatedly beat him "in the name of god." When she hit him, usually with a belt across his back, she screamed that she was doing it so he could be good, so that he would be seen favorably in the eyes of god. Working with the internalized messages and shame, without negating the presence of god in this boy's mind, was a challenge. Thankfully he was moved to a foster home where he was not abused.

Also while living in the south, I observed that patriarchy was alive and well. Many of my clients lived in extended family systems with the grandfather seen as the wise, respected elder. I remember one girl's mother was certain it would be pointless to bring her father into a family session because he did not believe in therapy and he would not interact with me (a young woman). I arranged for us to play a game that I often use in the beginning stages of family treatment (Talking, Feeling, Doing game – Creative Therapeutics), and I invited grandpa to sit at the head of the table (to maintain his sense of being in control). He was encouraged to join us but told he did not have to. As the family began playing, he periodically interjected or commented playfully on a member's game response, eventually sliding over to his grandson's side. With the pressure off, he joined the game part way through. Though he was not able to "buy in" to therapy or share any emotional content during the game, he was able to join us because I joined with him in a nonthreatening way.

Another case that comes to mind was that of a 12-year-old Muslim boy. He was a gifted youngster who had been physically abused by his mother and he was living in foster care when he came to treatment. As a dog lover, I often use my love of animals to explore and connect early in treatment. My young client appeared puzzled that I would love dogs so much. He went on to explain that dogs are only used for guarding and hunting within his culture, and he thought they were gross, dirty beasts. I had never heard this before so, rather than being shocked by his perspective, I did some research to understand the Muslim view of dogs. I also had to ensure my young client had a private space for his late afternoon prayer (asr) since his appointments were usually at 5pm and late afternoon prayers were done shortly after 5pm. Additionally, I noticed that when his mother and stepfather joined us for family sessions, his stepfather was very distant (physically) when greeting, while his mother shook my hand. I later learned that there are cultural gender norms.

Some religions do not celebrate birthdays. I learned this when working with a young girl raised by Jehovah Witness parents. So when I began working with her, I was mindful to not include birthday celebration analogies. For example, when youth are taught breathing activities, one of them involves smelling the flower (inhale through your nose) and blow out the birthday candles (exhale through the mouth).

Finally, during the assessment process, it is important that we do not assume heterosexuality. As noted in Chapter 3's Time Line activity, we ask about significant others rather than asking gendered questions (e.g. Do you have a boyfriend? Or, when was your first girlfriend?). Ask your client what pronoun(s) they prefer to use as well.

6. Use a Strength-Focused, Collaborative Approach

Despite the inherent power differential in the therapeutic relationship, compounded for youth with little to no choice in the decision to attend therapy, we must provide a collaborative approach. This means that children and youth are part of the treatment planning process, and we want to select interventions based on their interests and strengths. Incorporating interests and strengths provides opportunities for mastery and fosters a sense of empowerment. Collaborative approaches include therapist attunement, movement at the client's pace, encouragement of mindful curiosity and exploration, and we typically offer abundant psychoeducation throughout the treatment process (Ogden, Minton & Pain, 2006). A collaborative approach helps us ensure that the client understands what we are doing and why, rather than having them blindly follow along. This is especially important with traumatized youth who may never have had a voice or choice.

Note that sometimes we have to use our clinical judgment in a way that overrules the collaborative process. Following is a brief example:

> I was working with an 18-year-old girl who had a horrific history of abuse. She had limited memory of her childhood trauma. As always, I prefaced an experiment with acknowledgment of the possibility that she could be triggered, and I reminded her that she could stop at any time with a hand signal or word. We were working on finding ways to give her a sense of grounding as she tended to dissociate and had little body awareness. I introduced the idea of rolling her foot over a supple, spiky ball, and then I demonstrated the movement. As my client began moving her foot over the ball, she recalled that she had read a medical report that described severe injuries to her feet. She indicated that she had no memory of the injuries but did recall the report. I suggested we stop the activity, but my client insisted she could practice this at home because she had no recollection of the incidents other than what she read in the report. This was a point to provide additional psychoeducation about trauma living in the body and the potential to trigger a dissociative state with this particular activity was explored. We agreed that this was not an ideal grounding exercise.

7. Meet the Client Where They're at

Clinicians must strive to match their clients energetically. This may involve mirroring movement, monitoring and adjusting eye gaze or head position, and initially matching and then shifting our prosody. For example, if our client is sitting curled in the corner of the sofa, her eyes cast downward and she is verbally unresponsive, we are not going to encourage a felt sense of safety by speaking in a fast-paced, high-pitched tone. Meet the client where she is, offer her space and a calm presence. Conversely, if you have a client who cannot sit still and is highly activated and hyperverbal, speaking to him in a soft, calm tone is not going to get us any traction. Match his arousal, engage him in playful activities while slowly titrating to bring him to a place inside his window of tolerance where he can be present and comprehend what is happening in the session.

Extremely important with adolescents – be authentic! Children have excellent radar and will call us out if they sense we are being disingenuous. Demonstrate, through your actions and words, what Adlerians call the "courage to be imperfect" (Dreikurs, 1991, p. 38). Modeling this for caregivers is important as well. Without being self-deprecating, find opportunities (such as with the Body Feelings Map, detailed in Chapter 8) to model the acceptance of imperfection. Traumatized and attachment-disordered youth may have learned that the only way to receive necessary love and nurturing is to be perfect. Their sense of worth is contingent on identifying and meeting another's needs. Their non-verbal narratives will reflect this. For example, we may observe a pulling back of the body or averted gaze as a youth responds to a question or engages in an activity. We may sense hesitation or fear, hypothesizing that he experienced abuse or ridicule for making a mistake, or not getting it right, in similar situations in the past. We can offer them examples of being okay, not being perfect, and being accepted just as we are.

8. Developmentally Appropriate Interventions vs. Age-Based

Perry (in Malchiodi & Crenshaw, 2014, p. 186) states: "The key to treatment is that the child is regulated and that relational and cognitive expectations are appropriate for the child's developmental age." If we utilize interventions geared for a particular age group and we are working with a child with a history of profound neglect, for example, we may fall short in meeting that child's needs. Mateo, discussed elsewhere throughout this book, is an example of an adolescent for whom I often had to consider interventions more appropriate for a latency-aged child.

9. Titration and Scaffolding

We want to engender competence and confidence in our youth. One way to do that is to provide activities that allow them to succeed. Success is motivating. We may be working with a child who has never felt he could measure up. As a result, we may see a young man who is constantly overcompensating, or we may see a young man who gives up easily or refuses to try something new. In the education world, scaffolding is used to help motivate children to achieve. A simple example might be teaching students to read and enunciate individual words before learning to read a complete sentence. If she succeeds with the words, she is going to feel more motivated to try full sentences. In the therapy world, titration is a similar concept. For example, if we learn that a girl is being verbally abused by her brother, we would not suggest that she go home and set a firm, clear boundary with him as a first step. First, we might explore her understanding of boundaries, her experience of setting a boundary (verbally or physically) through her core organizers (5-sense perception, thoughts, emotions, movement and sensation). We might then experiment with setting and embodying boundaries that feel right to her. Titration is a central feature of Sensorimotor Psychotherapy™ as we recognize that youth with complex trauma can shoot out of their windows of tolerance quickly (Ogden, 2015). We dip our toes in a little at a time, returning to a place of calm and safety. This expands the window of tolerance and allows the child to see that she can manage small amounts of distress without being overwhelmed. Too much too soon can be overwhelming and send a child outside their window of tolerance, possibly causing further dysregulation and decompensation.

10. Play!

It is important for us to be creative and playful in our work with traumatized youth. Play is different for young children than it is for adolescents, and there are also developmental considerations, so we must be mindful of the interventions we use (Gaskill & Perry, in Malchiodi & Crenshaw, 2014). Play lends itself nicely to somatic methods because it is movement-based, can be multisensory, and play often encourages exploration of relationship to the self and others. Youth who have experienced trauma or neglect may have never experienced the spontaneity and joy of play. As Ogden and Fisher (2007) assert: "Playfulness cannot develop in the shadow of threat and danger, a fact that carries debilitating and far-ranging consequences characteristic of the plight of traumatized individuals." (p. 1). We see incompatibility with play in the freeze response: rigid body, orientation to threat, racing heart and held breath. With the fight response, there is no possibility of play. In order for play to occur, according to Polyvagal Theory, the myelinated social engagement branch needs to be activated so that it can dampen the activated sympathetic nervous system (Rosenberg, 2017).

Yet we are hard-wired to play: Jaak Panksepp (aka The Rat Tickler) conducted ground-breaking research revealing the intrinsic nature of play (Panksepp, 2003; Panksepp, 2010). While I am not in favor of animal research, I giggle every time I watch Panksepp's fascinating research videos (see, for example, youtu. be/j-admRGFVNM and youtu.be/ieP3lpyOHtU). Despite play being natural to children around the world, Gray (2011) decries the decline in play in the present day. He correlates reduction in play with an increase in child psychopathology.

So how do we reestablish the propensity for play in our young traumatized clients? We need to be cognizant of the possibility that play was used in the grooming or perpetration of sexual abuse; thus play may take on a different meaning, one fraught with shame. Play is not a safe activity for these youth. As with anything else, let the youth take the lead. Play challenges habitual responses (Ogden, 2017): we can observe the child's patterns and slowly (remember titration) introduce playful activities that elicit opposite responses. For example, the child with arms held tightly at her side might initially have difficulty catching and rolling a ball back, but we can experiment in a playful, nonthreatening way that, through repetition and rhythm, develops that capacity. Play may not be possible until the youth has stabilized, has an expanded window of tolerance, and is capable of returning to his window through either self- or co-regulation activities. We might then introduce play through tossing a ball or engaging in the scribble game (a coloring activity where one person draws a scribble and the other person expands the scribble while creating a story), or we might invite them to play with the sand tray. Again, we base our considerations on the youth's interests and strengths.

11. Psychoeducation

Psychoeducation is a central feature to somatic methods in trauma treatment (Blaustein & Kinneburgh, 2010; Ogden & Fisher, 2015). Although it serves many purposes, one of the key goals of psychoeducation is to reduce the sense of shame, confusion, and "craziness" clients tend to feel. We might help a young client explore the sudden freeze response she gets whenever a man stands close to her on the subway, for example. As we explore what it was like to grow up with an intrusive father, we might notice the freeze response emerge in the room as widened eyes, holding of the breath, paling of the skin, and tautness of the body. We might contact what we see and, depending on how dysregulated she is, deepen the experience to uncover the thoughts and feelings associated with her present moment sensations. Once stabilized or grounded, we can discuss how her body has a natural reaction to a situation that was scary. I often use white boards to draw brain models, and Janina Fisher's flip charts to help normalize and validate client's present day response to past trauma.

Psychoeducation can occur prior to an activity, such as prefacing experiments and/or interventions with acknowledgment of the possibility that the client could be triggered, that particular activities are not for everyone, and a reminder that the client is free to stop at any time. For example, I was working with an adolescent on grounding. I introduced and demonstrated one method by rolling the sole of my foot over a small spiky ball. The client noted that they have no memory of what happened, but that she read a police report about her feet being punctured and infected. My client attempted to assure me that she was okay to practice the activity at home because she had no recollection of what the report referred to; however, I reminded her that trauma lives in the body and there is potential for her to trigger something through this activity.

We must also educate caregivers about the trauma response and ways to help their child move back into the window of tolerance. SMART (Warner et al., 2012) includes the caregivers in treatment, and the framework offers many opportunities to provide psychoeducation in the moment with youth. Contacting (therapist names what she sees) and modeling can play roles in psychoeducation. SMART helps caregivers recognize and track the signs (movement, cognitive processes, emotional regulation) of dysregulation. I use laminated charts so that we can circle the signs for the individual child, and the caregiver can track and intervene when she recognizes that the child is above or below his window of tolerance. Of course, psychoeducation about the impact of trauma on a child is important to reduce guilt and shame that the caregiver may feel.

12. Self-Care, Compassion Fatigue, Vicarious Trauma, and Burnout

Self-care is a critical, often overlooked factor in working effectively with traumatized people. Clinicians working with traumatized youth and families are especially susceptible to negative repercussions of trauma work (Abendroth & Figley 2013; Hyatt-Burkhart, 2014; Osofsky, 2011). As Osofsky (2011) asserts: "All professionals working with young traumatized children need to find individual ways to gain support and reduce the risk of ongoing VT to ensure that their work is effective and helpful." (p. 347). My intention was to offer a few paragraphs about this topic; however, as I began writing, I reflected on how often the topic is neglected in trauma books and workshops, and the significance of covering this material in depth for clinicians working with traumatized youth.

Compassion Fatigue, Vicarious Trauma, and Burnout

Compassion fatigue (CF), vicarious trauma (VT), and burnout are often used interchangeably. While there is considerable overlap in symptoms, the conditions comprise different risk factors and may manifest differently in helping professionals (e.g. child protection workers, psychotherapists, psychologists, nurses, social workers, first responders). CF and VT are also referred to as secondary traumatic stress since they arise from (prolonged, chronic) exposure to the trauma of others. Mathieu (2012) defines CF as "the profound emotional and physical erosion that takes place when helpers are unable to refuel and regenerate...VT describes the transformation of our view of the world due to cumulative exposure to traumatic images or stories." (p. 14). As Pearlman and Caringi (in Courtois & Ford, 2009) note, helpers' VT responses often parallel those of complex trauma survivors in terms of emotional, psychological, cognitive, and interpersonal disturbances. Figley (2017) expands on the definition of CF as a "reduced capacity or interest in being empathic or bearing the suffering of clients" (p. 2). Jirek (2015) added the dimension of "soul pain" to reflect the provider's spiritual unrest and anger at the state of the world. Cumulative, prolonged, and chronic are key in VT and CF, just as they are in the development of C-PTSD in clients. Van Dernoot Lipsky's (2009) book identifies a multiplicity of consequences of the "trauma exposure response," encompassing symptoms of both CF and VT; furthermore, she clarifies the difference between a typical hard day at work and the effects of trauma exposure: bone-tired, heart-tired, soul-tired exhaustion.

"Pain and suffering is all around us; it's not just at work. Where do we draw the line?" (Mathieu, 2012, p. 48). This question resonates with most of us who work with traumatized children and families. We encounter situations daily where we have to decide whether to intervene or walk away. It is difficult to switch off the propensities that drew us to this work in the first place.

Burnout refers to the sense of overwhelm one might feel due to stressors in the workplace such as competing demands, high caseload, and lack of management support. Burnout can occur in any occupation, while CF and VT tend to occur in occupations where there is cumulative exposure to the traumatic experiences of others. Perry (2014) and Figley (2002) note that "the cost of caring" can be detrimental to providers as well as clients. A clinician may experience CF, VT, or burnout separately or in combination. It is ironic that stigma surrounds experiencing or talking about personal mental health issues that may arise while performing the very work that increases vulnerability to be profoundly emotionally and psychologically impacted. Clinicians may feel embarrassed or weak, or they might worry that their supervisors judge their work performance negatively. Following are some of the signs and symptoms, risk factors, and practices to mitigate or prevent VT, CF, or burnout.

Risk Factors

- working conditions: lack of peer support, unmanageable caseload, lack of autonomy/control in the workplace, inadequate supervision, chaotic/ unstable or toxic work environment;
- excessive stress in personal life, illness, or family;
- lack of training (e.g. lack of trauma-specific training);
- insufficient self-care and work/home balance;
- lack of self-awareness/capacity for self-reflection.

For in-depth discussion of risk factors for VT and CF, see Mathieu (2012), Osofsky (2011), Abendroth and Figley (2013), Hyatt-Burkhart (2014), and Middleton and Potter (2015).

Signs and Symptoms

Signs and symptoms of VT (e.g. Mathieu, 2012; Sprang, Clark & Whitt-Woosley, 2007):

- inability to stop thinking about a client/clients;
- intrusive imagery or thoughts about clients' traumas;
- PTSD symptoms such as avoidance, hypervigilance, increased startle response;
- altered world view;
- decreased self-care;
- sadness, depression, despair;
- social withdrawal;
- detachment;
- increased physical complaints and illness;
- nightmares/sleep disturbance;
- self-medication with alcohol or drugs;
- emotional numbing;
- interruptions in sense of safety, trust, and intimacy.

Signs and symptoms of CF (e.g. Figley, 2002; Figley and Figley, 2017; Mathieu, 2012):

- anger and irritability;
- emotional lability;
- physical exhaustion;
- somatic symptoms (e.g. headaches, migraines, compromised immune system);
- decreased capacity for empathy and compassion;
- difficulty setting limits and boundaries;
- avoiding difficult topics with clients;
- discouragement, helplessness;
- feelings of incompetence;
- loss of separation between personal and professional lives.

Signs and symptoms of burnout (e.g. Jirek, 2015; Krasner et al., 2009; Sprang, Clark & Whitt-Woosley, 2007):

- absenteeism;
- impaired clinical judgment;
- low motivation;
- poor quality and productivity;
- friction among staff;
- emotional numbing;
- cynicism;
- feelings of dissatisfaction;
- decreased ability to empathize or care;
- high staff turnover (organizational indicator).

There are obvious costs to providers experiencing VT, CF, or burnout. The corollary of high staff turnover is longer wait lists for young traumatized clients and families. Early intervention saves the youth from years of distressing symptoms and may prevent entrenchment of maladaptive coping skills and, as demonstrated by ACEs research, is cost-effective. Most importantly, blurred boundaries or poor quality of care can harm clients. Everall and Paulson (2004) note the inevitable consequences of doing clinical work, but highlight the importance of mitigating the risk of secondary traumatic stress (VT or CF) to prevent violation of ethical principles. A study by Middleton and Potter (2015) found that child welfare professionals with higher rates of VT were more likely to leave the workplace. Ultimately, clinicians experiencing VT, CF, or burnout may leave the field and we lose caring, skilled mental health providers.

Knowing Your "Red Zone"

Mathieu (2012) uses a traffic light metaphor to illustrate the progression of CF and VT, noting that most of us live in the yellow zone most of the time. Further, Mathieu normalizes the experience of being in the edge of the red zone as "a normal consequence of doing a good job" (p. 48). It is essential that we familiarize ourselves with our yellow and red zone indicators so that we can make adjustments to mitigate CF and VT. In *The Compassion Fatigue Workbook*, Mathieu also reviews the components of four steps to wellness:

1. Take stock of stressors (at home and in the workplace).
2. Identify ways to enhance self-care and achieve work/life balance.
3. Develop skills to increase resilience (e.g. relaxation and stress management).
4. Commit to implementing changes.

There are many ways we can monitor and manage our state, but we must also recognize that there are levels beyond the individual that can prevent the development of CF/VT (e.g. organizational, systems). When I give workshops or consultations, I often refer to Mathieu's traffic light metaphor to illustrate the importance of clinicians monitoring their own state, and to encourage them to explore ways to manage their wellness on an ongoing basis.

Protective and Mitigating Factors

Osofsky (2011) has identified two levels involved in the prevention and recognition of VT: organizational and individual. We can advocate for wellness programs, adequate supervision, and opportunities to debrief with peers within our organizations. I have been fortunate to have worked at organizations that provided buffers and supports, such as wellness rooms to rest and recharge, leadership opportunities on committees, recognition and encouragement of mental health days off, and skilled supervision; conversely, I have worked with organizations that offered minimal support, pathologized trauma therapists' distress that led to depression or PTSD symptoms, self-medication and, ultimately, departure from the agency. Mathieu (2012) notes the importance of debriefing opportunities but cautions against sharing the horrific, graphic details of client trauma, a process Mathieu aptly calls "sliming" (p. 43). Venting and sharing are helpful to return a triggered or distressed clinician, but it is not necessary or helpful that the details of a client's traumatic experience be shared. Adequate, regular supervision is a protective factor for CF, VT, and burnout, but especially important for VT. Supportive, skilled supervisors can help clinicians recognize that they are heading toward a state of VT and can implement protective measures, such as normalization of the experience of VT when working with traumatized youth, suggest specific training or time off, or recommend additional supports such as psychotherapy if needed. Perry (2014) reminds us of the importance of maintaining work/life balance, and he recommends that we reclaim our sense of joy and meaning by spending time with emotionally healthy children. We can certainly develop a skewed perspective about children by spending so much time with traumatized youth. Coping strategies, healthy exercise, nutrition, and sleep habits are protective factors and something clinicians have control over.

CF can often be mitigated by ensuring the clinician's caseload is manageable, and mixing it up so that there are a variety of presenting issues. For example, having a few youth with presenting concerns such as social anxiety or ADHD can offset the impact of constant empathic engagement with complexly traumatized youth and families. Perry (2014) suggests that self-awareness and staying emotionally healthy and motivated thwart the onset of CF. Salston and Figley (2003) emphasize that, left unchecked, secondary traumatic stress (CF) can lead to secondary traumatic stress disorder (VT). Detachment and a sense of achievement have also been identified as a protective factor for CF (Figley, 2003). Ironically, the capacity to empathically engage makes us effective in our work, but we must also be able to maintain a degree of detachment in order to remain effective. Figley (2017) notes that providers frequently fail to maintain self-care basics that are essential to work/life balance, and he identifies five protective factors: nutrition, rest/sleep, social support, physical exercise, and engaging in activities that give a sense of joy. As with VT, social support is a protective factor for CF: clinicians constantly exposed to clients' traumatic stories withdraw and feel alienated from friends and family because they sense that they do not share or understand their world view. Maintaining connections to people who do not work in the field is important to balance, just as regular access to peer supports and supervision is protective. Compassion satisfaction is considered an antidote to compassion fatigue and burnout (Osofsky, 2011). Finally, checklists, such as the ProQOL, can help us monitor our level of CF. The literature identifies a range of protective factors against burnout, most notably organizational support, ongoing training opportunities, autonomy in the workplace, and manageable caseloads (Perry, 2014; Sprang, Clark & Whitt-Woosley, 2007).

ProQOL: Professional Quality of Life Self-Test

The ProQOL, developed by Stamm in 2009 and revised in 2012, is a self-scoring assessment of the presence of burnout, compassion fatigue, and compassion satisfaction. Whether I am giving a workshop or providing clinical consultation to mental health professionals, this is one of the first things we talk about. In addition to the self-scoring form, there is an app (developed by the National Center for Telehealth and Technology – a link to the app is given in the appendices) clinicians can download, and their scores can be tracked over time. The app includes various helpful tools, such as physical exercises that can be done seated or standing throughout the workday, and tips to enhance resilience. When working with other clinicians, I recommend that they complete the self-test every three to six months and make changes to have more work/life balance, or seek support if needed.

Vicarious Post-traumatic Growth (VPTG)

Hyatt-Burkhart (2014) advocates that we shift from a deficit-based approach to a focus on the positive effects of working with traumatized children and adolescents. As with a client's post-traumatic growth, defined as the positive change and personal growth following a traumatic experience, there is possibility for change and personal growth following clinician trauma exposure. Post-traumatic growth can be evaluated with clients, and measures, such as the Posttraumatic Growth Inventory (available at www.emdrhap.org/content/wp-content/uploads/2014/07/VIII-B_Post-Traumatic-Growth-Inventory.pdf), can be adapted for clinicians to monitor their VPTG. Proponents of VPTG note that recognition of positive, growth-inducing effects of traumatic experiences is not meant to negate the negative effects. Tedeschi and Calhoun (1996) developed the Post-traumatic Growth Inventory to assess the potential benefits (e.g. improved relationships with others, changed self-perception and meaning of life) from having gone through a traumatic event.

Your Own Therapy

It is irresponsible and unethical for clinicians to address their unresolved issues in their clinical work. As clinicians, we may be triggered and can experience

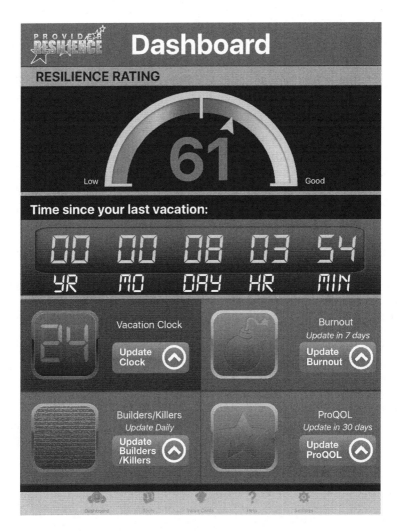

Figure 4.1 ProQOL App – Sample Screen Shot

countertransference in the therapeutic relationship. Additionally, we may have external stressors, such as financial challenges or an ill family member, which compound our susceptibility to VT or CF. Figley (2002) stresses the importance of seeking support to deal with our stress in order to effectively help our clients.

Supervision and Consultation

As noted above, the extent of CF and VT can be mitigated with regular opportunities to debrief with peers, and ongoing supervision. I currently meet with a monthly peer supervision group that focuses on trauma and dissociation, and I maintain monthly consultations with peers as well as a consulting mentor.

Illustration of VT and CF

Several years ago, I was working at a sexual assault center (SAC) two days per week, and I was also working at a children's mental health agency three days per week. Most of the clients at the SAC had horrific, complex trauma histories, and many were experiencing severe structural dissociation. The theory of structural dissociation, covered later in this book, was new to me. Thankfully, I had a competent, skilled clinical supervisor at the SAC. The women and men I saw at the SAC were also presenting with symptoms of complex trauma such as self-injury, suicidal ideation and behavior, addictions, and intergenerational trauma.

The perfect storm brewed with additional life stressors: a long commute to the SAC; I was in the midst of completing requirements for registration with a regulatory college and attending an intensive training program (Sensorimotor Psychotherapy™); and my beloved dog had recently died. The signs and symptoms of VT and CF that I began to experience included: physical and emotional exhaustion, irritability and lability, somatic symptoms (headaches/migraines, nausea) that led to an increase in sick days, sleep disturbance (insomnia, hypersomnia), isolation and social withdrawal, difficulty with concentration and memory, poor eating habits, an inability to separate work/personal life (thinking/ worrying about clients), and I dreaded seeing some clients. I had not hit this wall previously and it frightened me, eroded my sense of competence as a mental health professional: it was a wake-up call to improve my self-care and seek support when needed.

Although the SAC was supportive and supervision helped me recognize the need to alleviate the effects of the trauma exposure, paperwork and productivity demands did not change. I realized that I had to make changes in how I managed the work/life balance, and I needed to enhance my coping skills. To begin recuperating and recharging, I met with a stress management specialist who provided me with tools to improve my self-regulation skills, and she also provided auricular acupuncture. The latter was fascinating and I was impressed with how quickly the procedure lowered my stress response. Also, I began attending qigong and Nia classes, developed better eating habits and a regular bedtime routine, and I reconnected with friends for social interaction outside of the workplace. Finally, I reengaged in a variety of creative endeavors (e.g. drawing, painting, playing guitar). I began to monitor my stress levels on a regular basis and readjusted practices as needed.

5 Working with Systems

As we work with a child and his environment, the child starts to calm, experiences more regulated arousal, and becomes more aware of safety in his world.

(Sandra Wieland, 2017, p. 4)

The complexity of clinical work with children and adolescents involves not simply providing treatment for an individual. Our work is compounded by the fact that we often engage with myriad adults involved in the child's life. Thus, we must consider the child's many systems when striving toward enhancing regulatory capacity and a felt sense of safety. With younger children, more so than with adolescents, we are working in conjunction with systems:

- education (e.g. school, day care, therapeutic day treatment);
- child protection services;
- legal, police, courts, or juvenile justice providers;
- treatment funding agencies;
- previous or concurrent clinicians; other providers (e.g. pediatrician, psychiatrist);
- cultural/traditional/religious community;
- residential, respite, or foster care providers;
- the agency for whom we work;
- our regulatory/licensing bodies.

The above list is lengthy, and we have not even mentioned caregivers. Caregivers, as Wieland (2017) asserts, are our other clients. In her latest (and final) brilliant contribution to the field, *Parents Are Our Other Client*, she masterfully illustrates the intricacy of our involvement with our young client's caregiver(s). Through vignettes, Wieland elucidates the importance of clinicians attending to their own self-regulation (e.g. through centering, taking breaths), mentalization (i.e. thinking about thinking), and the need for attunement and validation of caregivers' experiences. As clinicians we can get caught up in our alliance with the youth to the detriment of effective treatment. We need to remember that we are working with caregivers who carry the legacy of their own trauma histories. Compassion, for the caregiver who is doing the best they can with what they have in this moment, and for ourselves as we notice that we are having a reaction to a caregiver's words or actions, will go a long way in the treatment of traumatized youth. More about working with caregivers appears in Chapter 7. Let us now turn to case vignettes that illustrate a few challenges we face in our work with our young clients' systems of care.

Case Illustrations

Vincent

As you may recall, Vincent was a 14-year-old boy who presented as anxious and depressed, and he was using substances to self-medicate. Given his previous hospitalizations and mental health providers, I requested consent from Vincent and his caregivers to allow information exchange and obtain reports. This was done through fax and email, and his mother also provided copies of records. Vincent had been referred by a victim services program for youth so his funding was limited. After a few sessions, Vincent disclosed that he had recently experienced sextortion (threats to share sexually compromising images via social media or text). Given the previous negative experiences with systems that left him feeling mistrustful and helpless, I knew it was essential that we follow through with reporting the incident. Of course, there are also mandated reporting requirements. The police were contacted and an officer came to take Vincent's statement. The officer was kind and supportive, and he reassured Vincent that he had done nothing wrong. This was reparative for Vincent. Afterward, Vincent appeared calmer and expressed relief that he was able to do something about the incident. Far too often police receive attention for their inappropriate behavior, so I thought that it was important to contact the officer's supervisor to share my client's positive experience.

Following the report, I contacted the funding agency. The disclosure was a discrete incident, and thus Vincent qualified for additional funding. I had collaborated with victim service agencies for years by then and found them to be supportive and understanding; there was no hesitation on their part to extend the funding. Subsequently, I joined his parents to advocate for victim's compensation. Not only had his parents taken time off from work to attend to their son's needs, but also there were expenses related to after-school care for his sister, and there were missteps that led to further deterioration and hospitalization. Vincent's earlier interaction with the police officer had instilled some trust and he was empowered to pursue justice. Many months later I attended a hearing with him, and I was horrified as the panelists grilled him about the assaults that occurred when he was only 12 years old. I had not previously attended a similar hearing and did not know what to expect, but they granted Vincent's request that I attend with him. I assumed they would be more understanding about the impact of his age, his mental state at the time of the assaults, and the time that had passed since the assaults (i.e. memory).

As the hearing ended, one panelist asked a question that flagrantly reflected his heterosexism; moreover, it appeared that he had not heard anything Vincent had said regarding his attraction to males. I noticed that Vincent appeared rattled and shut down, so I asked if he wanted me to respond. As he nodded, I answered the panelist's question while Vincent fidgeted with an object that he had brought with him to stay grounded. Following the hearing, I wrote a letter suggesting sensitivity and diversity training. Vincent reviewed and approved the letter before it was mailed.

Adele

Adele and her parents had seen a therapist prior to me to address family issues. Her referral to me was specifically to work on concerns related to internet exploitation. Interactions with her parents were cordial and they presented as committed to helping their daughter. Though Adele presented as outgoing, she was somewhat guarded when it came to exploration or expression of feelings. She often used humour to deflect her discomfort. Her parents were quite stoic so I knew that I would have to engage them around emotional awareness and expression to help Adele move forward in this area. When we learned that the police had uncovered additional incidents of exploitation, Adele shrugged it off. However, an increase in self-injurious behaviour and self-deprecating comments followed.

Since Adele's parents were not involved in her treatment regularly, I advised Adele that we needed to include them in creating a safety plan. She was hesitant about their involvement because, as she explained, they thought she had stopped cutting a year ago. She was also surprised I wanted to do anything because her previous therapist was aware of the cutting and did not involve the parents. By this time, Adele trusted me enough to permit the contact with her parents about safety planning. We did it together, with Adele's input and agreement at every step; in fact, she wrote her own safety plan that she subsequently shared with her teachers at school. The parents, and Adele, had previously signed a consent form to share information, so I contacted Adele's other therapist to inquire about the self-injury. It is imperative that providers be on the same page regarding treatment planning to avoid confusing the clients. I also felt it necessary to address the lack of concern, per Adele, about the cutting. We had a pleasant conversation and discovered that we were on the same page. When funding ended, I was happy to have spoken with the other therapist as Adele's parents ended treatment with me and returned to the other therapist to continue family work.

Mateo

Mateo was involved with multiple children's services agencies when I began working with him. Mateo was referred to my agency by child protection services and he started TF-CBT as part of a city-wide research project. The school had expressed concerns about his functioning and learning in the classroom so classroom visits were arranged. After observation, it was apparent that he would benefit from the agency's day treatment (school-based) program. In order to facilitate registration with the program, I attended plan-of-care meetings organized by the child protection service agency. These meetings included child protection service workers, representatives from the foster care system, a child and youth worker who was arranging assessment of FASD, and coordination with a social worker who provided weekly in-home meetings with his foster parents. After a couple of meetings, providers agreed that Mateo would enter the day treatment program and I would offer joint in-home sessions with the social worker. The social worker was integral since the foster parents primarily spoke Spanish.

Mateo's flat affect, sluggish movements, frequent daydreaming, impulsivity, and difficulty grasping academic material frustrated day treatment staff. Mateo spoke limited English at this point so communication was a challenge. He was often removed from the classroom, isolated from peers, and sometimes restrained by staff. One of the advantages of working within an agency with multiple programs is access to additional resources: Mateo was referred to the art therapist, and I also requested a psychoeducational assessment with our agency psychologist to determine whether Mateo had a learning disability. I increased his sessions to twice weekly as he was learning skills to regulate himself, to recognize and express his feelings in age-appropriate ways, and he was engaged in the activities offered in sessions. Learning to recognize and express his feelings in age-appropriate ways, especially with peers, was an important goal for Mateo as he often presented as younger due to developmental lags. Mateo did well one-on-one, and he was growing confident as his artistic skills progressed. He liked to share and repeat activities done with his art therapist. He began to smile and display an offbeat sense of humour. Sometimes Mateo asked school staff if he could meet with me, and this was perceived as manipulation. Mateo was often told to "use his words" when he had emotional or behavioral outbursts, but Mateo had limited English and he was likely in a dissociated or limbic state at the time. I was concerned about him because I was increasingly aware of how traumatized this youngster was and felt powerless to meet his treatment needs with so many providers and perspectives involved. Occasionally, I dropped into the school to check in on Mateo and after witnessing disturbing treatment of him, such as being restrained against a wall and being accused of lying and shamed in front of his peers, I requested a meeting with the program coordinator. We discussed the necessity of providing trauma-informed treatment to Mateo (and likely other youth involved with the program). In a previous agency where I was a clinical supervisor, I had witnessed the "us and them" climate that can manifest between program staff, such as child and family therapists and child and youth workers, and I was able to bring staff together for a workshop that clarified their positions and enhanced respect among staff. I offered to work with the staff to find ways to better track and understand his behavior and requested that the agency provide trauma-focused care training for all staff.

Unfortunately, Mateo decompensated and his adoptive parents placed him in a residential care program. His foster parents grew exasperated with his frequent lying, hoarding, and inability to follow through with directives. Once in the residential program, he was no longer able to attend the day treatment classroom and his involvement with our agency terminated. Despite the multitude of services in place for this youngster, his foster parents had not been prepared to manage a traumatized child with such complex needs.

Looking back, what could have been done differently with Mateo?

Situations changed rapidly for this youth. At the time, I knew little about FASD so it might have helped to invite an expert speaker to a treatment planning meeting. I could have found other ways to inform staff about the impact of trauma (relational and abuse-related) on behavior, cognition, emotions, etc., perhaps by offering a short video at a treatment planning meeting. Perhaps I could have found ways to incorporate his strengths and interests in the classroom: he loved animals and was gentle with them, he liked to draw and create crafts, and he enjoyed basketball (one-on-one, he did not do well in gym class). His foster family would have benefited from information and planning around adoption of a child raised in an orphanage. Because it was a kinship-based adoption, these caregivers did not receive much information or guidance prior to adoption.

Working Within an Organization

An agency or organization is a system of care in itself. When we provide services to young clients while we work for an organization, there are policies and procedures to follow. Additionally, there are usually other programs and services, such as in-home family support, day treatment (classroom-based services), art or music therapy, and group services to coordinate. Access to various programs and services has its benefits as well, though, as we are able to offer more holistic treatment for youth and families. Having worked on both sides of the border (Canada/US), I am aware of the challenges we face in providing effective clinical services to children and families, often with expectations around direct service hours, and keeping on top of record-keeping, case management, and coordination with other providers. Organizational and time management skills, and a good support system of colleagues, are essential to avoiding burnout. As noted earlier in Chapter 4, self-care is frequently overlooked and we must be mindful of our own states to prevent compassion fatigue and vicarious trauma. Thankfully, many agencies have wellness committees and wellness rooms for clinicians. One strategy I have found helpful is to join such committees, if they exist in the agency, to participate in the shaping of the program and to gain a sense of empowerment.

MVA Clinic – CBT Approach

Organizations may also have specific approaches that guide their assessment and treatment programs. For example, some agencies firmly believe in the efficacy of CBT, while some believe that play therapy is the only way to work with young children, and employed clinicians are expected to follow the agency's model. Some organizations have not yet adopted trauma-informed or focused services and interventions. It is important to know whether your approach and related values are in alignment with those of an organization or there can be conflict. I am remembering a time I did contract work with an MVA (motor vehicle accident) clinic. The clinic utilized primarily CBT interventions. While I use CBT at times, it is not my primary method for traumatized youth. The clinic was open to my use of creative and somatic methods with young clients. They were not, however, open to learning about these methods for use with other clients. This became a complication with shared clients as the other clinicians relied on the CBT model. A colleague had recently recommended Scaer's (2007) *The Body Bears the Burden*, and I was enthralled with the content's applicability to MVA clinical work. Not all people who experience a traumatic auto accident are traumatized; there are other things to consider such as early attachment relationships, boundaries (present or not), and abuse histories. Using CBT seems inadequate without addressing these underlying issues. Beyond my enthusiastic recommendation of the book, there was not much I could do to shift the organizational culture.

Other Considerations

In addition to adherence to organizational policies and procedures, we have rules and regulations from our licensing bodies. Most of us belong to a regulatory body, such as the College of Psychologists of Ontario (CPO), the National Board for Certified Counselors (NBCC), or the Ontario College of Social Workers and Social Service Workers (OCSWSSW). These regulatory bodies ensure that practitioners maintain ongoing education in the field (e.g. CEUs), that we follow a code of ethical conduct, that we practice in our areas of competence, and that we have professional liability insurance. The regulatory bodies are essential and their main mandate is to protect the public. Sometimes, however, there may be conflict between agency practices and the rules of conduct stipulated by the regulatory body. For example, my college (CPO) states that we cannot accept gifts from clients with more than token value. While working with clients in conjunction with other clinicians at agencies, I have had to cite this code when offered thank you gifts at the end of treatment. This can be especially difficult when the other clinician does not adhere to such a code, perhaps because their regulatory body does not stipulate these requirements, and the decline of the gift can be disheartening to the client. We can gracefully thank our clients for their kindness, while assuring them that our College does not permit acceptance of gifts from clients. Should there be time (i.e. if they offered the gift at a time other than the end of treatment), we might want to explore the significance of the offering in a subsequent session.

6 Misunderstood Children
Diagnostic Dilemmas

> Children exposed to maltreatment, family violence or loss of their caregivers often meet diagnostic criteria from the *Diagnostic and Statistical Manual for Mental Disorders*, fifth edition (DSM 5) , for depression, attention-deficit/hyperactivity disorder (ADHD), oppositional defiant disorder (ODD), conduct disorder, anxiety disorders, eating disorders, sleep disorders, communication disorders, separation anxiety disorder, and reactive attachment disorder.
>
> (Cook, et al., 2005)

Children and youth have often been labeled with a multitude of diagnoses by the time they reach my office. Multiple diagnoses may reflect the lack of a comprehensive trauma assessment, or there has been a lack of consideration of the far-reaching manifestations of early childhood trauma and neglect. Over the years, I have had to call children's protection services to report disclosures from youth who had previously disclosed their abuse to former therapists. While it is heartening that the youth are comfortable enough to share their stories within the first few sessions, it is disheartening to know that they had gone through other service providers who either did not ask the right questions or did not believe their stories. Additionally, the youth have frequently been prescribed unnecessary or unhelpful medications prior to our initial meeting. The American Academy of Child and Adolescent Psychiatry (AACAP, 2012) states: "Given that there is a limited evidence base for efficacy of psychotropic medications in young children, medication should be used conservatively in this group." (p. 15). Moreover, psychiatric medication can have a negative impact on growing minds and bodies. Per AACAP (2012), "Active pursuit of alternative interventions to medications are [*sic*] especially important when there are serious side effects that can occur, such as weight gain or movement disorders, especially when medicine is prescribed over an extended period of time." (p. 6). According to a recent Canadian study, more than a third of Canadians have suffered some kind of child abuse in their lives, and research is increasingly finding a dose-response relationship between the number of types of child abuse experienced and the likelihood for complex mental health conditions, including disturbances in affect regulation (Afifi et al., 2014; Anda et al., 2006; Cloitre et al., 2009).

Developmental Trauma Disorder (DTD), formulated by Bessel van der Kolk and a group of expert clinicians in 2005, attempts to capture the impact of self-regulatory deficits in youth with a history of complex trauma and attachment injury. As noted by Cook et al. (2005): "Complex trauma exposure results in a loss of core capacities for self-regulation and interpersonal relatedness." (p. 390). The DTD working group identified seven areas as domains of impairment for children with complex trauma histories:

1. attachment;
2. biology;
3. affect regulation;
4. dissociation;
5. behavioral control;
6. cognition;
7. self-concept.

Clearly, these domains impact the trajectory of development; thus earlier identification of the impairments might prevent the long-term, far-reaching consequences that are seen with untreated trauma (e.g. physical, emotional, and mental health issues identified in the ACEs study). Despite van der Kolk and the DTD work group's efforts, including extensive field studies, DTD was not included in the DSM-5 (*Diagnostic and Statistical Manual*) published in 2013.

Research on youth in juvenile justice finds that more than 50% of incarcerated youth have been exposed to six or more traumatic events, such as domestic violence and physical or sexual abuse (Abram, 2004). Furthermore, youth with histories of polyvictimization are likely to have multiple diagnoses attached to them. Some youth present with externalizing behaviors and may be given a diagnosis of ADHD (Attention Deficit Hyperactivity Disorder) to account for their inability to focus or their high activity level. Others may be diagnosed with ODD (Oppositional Defiant Disorder) due to their refusal to follow rules, outright defiance of authority, or aggression toward people or property. Internalizing behaviors, on the other hand, are directed inward. These youth may receive diagnoses such as Depressive Disorder due to their low mood, anxiety disorders (e.g. fear or avoidance of situations, things, or people), or somatoform disorders due to a tendency to be ill or frequent complaints of physical problems such as headaches or stomachaches. There seems to be a gender difference in the attribution of externalizing versus internalizing behavior diagnoses.

Now we will turn to a review of the characteristics often identified in the misdiagnosis of traumatized youth. We know through research, such as ACEs, that childhood trauma is prevalent, and we know that trauma can impact children in myriad ways. Refer to Figure 6.1 for an illustration of the many ways trauma manifests in children and youth.

Now we shall review criteria for PTSD and Complex PTSD (C-PTSD), and discuss similarities.

Complex PTSD

The DSM-5 added Complex PTSD to account for additional symptoms overlooked in PTSD diagnosis. In addition to criteria listed in the PTSD diagnosis

THE MANY WAYS TRAUMA MAY PRESENT IN CHILDREN AND ADOLESCENTS

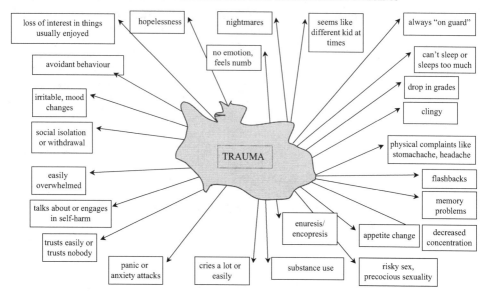

Figure 6.1 The Many Ways Trauma May Present in Youth

Source: Adapted from Janina Fisher, (2009). *Psychoeducational Aids for Working with Psychological Trauma.* Cambridge, MA: Kendall Press. www.janinafisher.com. Used with permission.

of the DSM IV-TR, Complex PTSD includes distorted perceptions of self, others, and the world (i.e. safety). Significantly, Complex PTSD was moved from the anxiety disorders section to the newly created trauma and stress-related disorders primarily because PTSD often manifests in symptoms that are not anxiety-related. Complex PTSD addresses trauma that is chronic and typically involves more than one type of trauma (e.g. sexual abuse, physical abuse, neglect, etc.). Below is a chart summarizing the similarities and differences. Note that these criteria apply to individuals who are older than 6 years of age. Additional criteria are applied for children under 6 years of age. Differences are noted in *italics*.

Complex PTSD	PTSD
Chronic/prolonged or multiple types of trauma, often of an interpersonal nature	*One or more time-limited* traumatic incident
Reexperiencing through intrusive thoughts, flashbacks, or nightmares	Reexperiencing through intrusive thoughts, flashbacks or nightmares
Avoidance of reminders of the trauma	Avoidance of reminders of the trauma
Hypervigilance or being "on guard" all the time	Hypervigilance or being "on guard" all the time
Affect dysregulation	
Problems with self-perception (negative self-concept including feelings of guilty and shame)	
Difficulties with interpersonal relationships	

The DSM-5 requires that many criteria are met in order to diagnose someone with C-PTSD (Criterion A through H) and there are two additional specifications (Dissociative: Depersonalization, Derealization, and Delayed). The details for the DSM-5 criteria can be found in the manual or online. Dissociation is the subject of Chapter 12 in this book. For preschool children (under 6 years of age), the DSM-5 has added a diagnostic subcategory under PTSD.

Another diagnostic resource is the ICD-11 (International Classification of Diseases, version 11). Some clinicians prefer to use the ICD, particularly those living and practicing outside of the United States. The DSM is published by the American Psychiatric Association, and the ICD is published by WHO (World Health Organization). Within Canada, I have used both sources for coding purposes, depending on the agency that I worked for. The most recent version of the ICD, ICD-11 released in June 2018, contains a diagnostic category for complex post-traumatic disorder. Note that the ICD classifies many conditions, not just psychiatric disorders (e.g. disorders of the immune system, diseases of the visual system). The ICD-11 user guide and coding tools are available free-of-charge online. For reference purposes, here is the description for complex post-traumatic stress disorder, retrieved from ICD online:

6B41 Complex post-traumatic stress disorder

Complex post-traumatic stress disorder (Complex PTSD) is a disorder that may develop following exposure to an event or series of events of an extremely threatening or horrific nature, most commonly prolonged or repetitive events from which escape is difficult or impossible (e.g., torture, slavery, genocide campaigns, prolonged domestic violence, repeated childhood sexual or physical abuse). The disorder is characterized by the core symptoms of PTSD; that is, all diagnostic requirements for PTSD have been met at some point during the course of the disorder. In addition, Complex PTSD is characterized by 1) severe and pervasive problems in affect regulation; 2) persistent beliefs about oneself as diminished, defeated or worthless, accompanied by deep and pervasive feelings of shame, guilt or failure related to the traumatic event; and 3) persistent difficulties in sustaining relationships and in feeling close to others. The disturbance causes significant impairment in personal, family, social, educational, occupational or other important areas of functioning.

(Retrieved June 2018 from icd.who.int/browse11/l-m/en#/
http://id.who.int/icd/entity/585833559)

As Cloitre (2015) notes, we can see different presentations (symptoms) in clients assigned the same diagnostic label, reducing the usefulness of labels for communication purposes. Moreover, as Smith (2007) asserts, widely used measures such as the CBCL (Child Behavior Checklist) and self-report questionnaires and assessment tools tend to capture "quantification of a perception" (p. 139). While more information about a child's functioning is advantageous to assessment and treatment, there are challenges to using multiple informants. For example, the rater is assessing the child in a particular setting (e.g. the classroom), and observations are based on the rater's thoughts and feelings about that particular child. It is interesting when diverse raters produce discrepant profiles that seem like they rated a completely different child. I have often seen hugely discrepant ratings from separated or divorced caregivers. Research on rater effects demonstrates a strong connection between caregiver (maternal) depression and psychopathology and elevated ratings of child behavior problems (Smith, 2007). Youth self-report inventories are useful as well, though they may also provide a clinical picture that is dissimilar from that of their caregiver's. Reasons for differences may include lack of self-awareness, denial of severity of problems, or exaggeration of severity of problems. Several assessment tools have built-in validity indicators to capture the possibility of a youth faking good or faking bad. Faking good and faking bad are indicators of under- or overreporting, respectively. Again, the purpose for the evaluation and motivation of the youth (e.g. mandated vs. voluntary treatment) play a role in the endorsement of items in self-report inventories.

So, what do we do with all of this confusing information? Psychometric tools are not stand-alone, even when there are multiple informants. The clinical interviews in various configurations of the family unit (e.g. child individually, child with caregiver 1, caregiver 1 individually, child with caregiver 2 and siblings, etc.) are most illuminating, and I use the information provided from ratings as supplemental material. Some clients find the visual output, such as graphs, useful especially when administered to assess progress throughout treatment. Diagnoses from previous clinicians may offer a starting point and I may request consent to share information with a former provider, but I always inform clients that I work with what is in front of me. I often give examples of how diagnoses, such as Generalized Anxiety, may present quite differently in people. Some clients request formal assessments and a diagnosis, usually when they are seeking documentation with a specific purpose (e.g. to obtain access to accommodation or support for academic or work settings).

Case Illustrations

Mateo

Mateo's presentation was confusing to the many professionals who worked with him, and frustrating to his family. At times Mateo was cheerful, but mostly he was quiet and appeared tuned-out from his surroundings. Also, he was prone to sudden aggressive outbursts. Staff and family members could not identify precipitating events or triggers to his rage episodes. He was less inclined to have outbursts at home; however, his frequent food hoarding and lying baffled his adoptive caregivers. Despite being placed with a loving, nurturing family, Mateo was unable to connect to others or regulate his affect. By the time Mateo and his family reached my agency, he had a host of diagnoses including RAD (Reactive Attachment Disorder), ODD (Oppositional Defiant Disorder), OCD (Obsessive Compulsive Disorder), Intermittent Explosive Disorder, and Bipolar I Disorder. Other diagnoses being queried were FASD (Fetal Alcohol Spectrum Disorder), learning disabilities, and developmental delays. That is a lot of diagnoses for an 11-year-old!

Given Mateo's first five years, I wondered about the possibility of trauma and neglect (in the orphanage). From a trauma perspective, many of his behaviors and symptoms made sense to me. Mateo presented with numerous symptoms of complex trauma: dysregulated affect, he reported (and drew) recurrent nightmares, he reported (and drew) incidents of physical and sexual assault that took place at the orphanage during the first five years of his life, he viewed himself as "bad," he was unable to engage in age-appropriate peer interactions, and he constantly seemed to be on guard while lost in a world of his own. Mateo did not feel safe connecting to others because his earliest relationships were fraught with pain, betrayal, and unmet needs. In fact, Mateo did not know what his needs were. It was like he was existing on autopilot, and it often seemed like there was nobody present inside.

From a trauma-informed perspective, we have to ask what happened to you, not what is wrong with you or why are you doing (behavior)? Mateo was experiencing the sequelae of developmental trauma, as well as other forms of trauma, that impeded his capacity to regulate across domains. In fact, his neurodevelopment was likely impeded by his early experiences. Behavioral interventions and talk therapy were not going to be effective for Mateo. First and foremost, he required safety, consistency, and predictability across settings, including school, social, and home. While his caregivers provided nurturance, they were not looking through a trauma lens and they saw his behavior as intentional. Psychoeducation for caregivers included helping them realize that Mateo learned ways to survive in his early environment and the strategies he learned became habituated response patterns. Shaming and blaming only served to increase his self-view as "bad." While Mateo had to learn that he was responsible for his whole self, an understanding of dissociative processes in youth would benefit school staff and caregivers. Calming reassurance would go further than restraints or raised voices and angry expressions with this youngster.

Mateo's situation reflects a failure in systems to meet a highly traumatized youth's needs, primarily because the people and programs involved were not aware, let alone skilled in working with complex trauma and dissociation. As work with this client occurred over a decade ago, I am hopeful that systems, organizations, and childcare professionals have furthered their understanding and skills in complex trauma. Based on conversations with colleagues in the field, and resources available online for organizational training, it appears we have moved in that direction.

Vincent

After two hospitalizations and clinical assessments, Vincent had received multiple diagnoses: Brief Psychotic Disorder, Major Depressive Disorder, Cannabis Use Disorder, and Generalized Anxiety Disorder. The diagnoses were given based on his behaviors over preceding months, including social isolation, fear of leaving the house, truancy, increase in use of cannabis, bouts of sadness and irritability, sleep and appetite disturbances, loss of interest in previously enjoyed activities, self-injury, onset of somatic complaints, and the presence of voices telling him to harm himself. Vincent had been prescribed various medications but he stopped taking them on his own without medical consultation because he did not like the side effects. Given Vincent's presenting symptoms, the diagnoses might have made sense; however, there was pertinent information that Vincent did not share because he was not asked the questions.

The consecutive sexual assaults that Vincent experienced resulted in classic PTSD symptoms (avoidance, intrusive images, memories and nightmares, heightened arousal and reactivity, and negative alterations in mood and cognitions about himself and a sense of safety in the world). Vincent attempted to cope with his distress by self-medicating and social withdrawal. He avoided situations and places that reminded him of the assaults, as he was frequently triggered into flashbacks, yet he also felt compelled to reenact (van der Kolk, 1989) and was subsequently revictimized. After he reenacted or engaged in similar activities that culminated in the sexual assaults, Vincent was filled with shame and self-loathing. The shame started a negative spiral of hopelessness and despair that were not mitigated by substance use. Vincent felt alone and disgusted in himself because he was gay, and he believed that he deserved the bad things that happened to him because he was bad. He grew suicidal, heard voices that told him to end his life, and he eventually attempted to take his life.

Vincent met the criteria for Complex PTSD because, in addition to the PTSD criteria, his trauma was interpersonal in nature, there were multiple incidents over a short period of time, he was severely dysregulated, and his perceptions of himself and the world were negatively impacted. The cumulative impact caused Vincent to split off parts of himself, feelings and thoughts and memories that he could not tolerate. His increasing self-hatred and shame manifested in angry, self-destructive tendencies (including voices that told him to kill himself). Vincent did not feel safe enough to share his assault history or sexual orientation with the mental health professionals that he encountered. Although he had a good relationship with his parents, he was terrified to tell them what had happened to him. As he was rejecting himself, he assumed that his parents would also reject him.

Through clinical interviews and psychometrics, we developed a treatment plan to address Vincent's many trauma symptoms. Safety and stabilization were paramount. Vincent was motivated to feel better and return to his previous level of functioning. He indicated that he felt understood by the therapist (me), and he was forthcoming with his experiences and the far-reaching impact they had on him. Vincent's thoughts and feelings, his impulses and behaviors were validated and normalized. He quickly learned to track his physiological responses and developed a variety of resources to return to the window of tolerance when triggered or otherwise dysregulated. He gained an understanding of the survival resources that he had developed to manage his overwhelming distress. Vincent's sleep improved, he reconnected with his family and friends, academic performance returned to its previous level, his assertiveness and ability to set boundaries increased, and the thoughts of self-harm dissipated. His eating-related and body issues continued for some time as his shame and self-loathing were directly connected to his perception of his body. Recognition of the purpose of his survival resources, such as cannabis use, social isolation, and self-injury, calmed Vincent's fears of being "crazy" and alleviated the profound sense of shame and guilt he carried around with him.

Vincent may have had a co-morbid depressive or anxiety disorder, and he was certainly self-medicating with cannabis, but his symptoms reflected the profound impact of complex trauma. When symptoms are understood as predictable sequelae of traumatic experiences, we can be more effective in planning and implementing treatment interventions; thus we can help the youth return to their developmental trajectories.

Dee

14-year-old Dee was considered oppositional at home and school. She engaged in self-injurious behaviors, substance use (weed) regularly, and she was prone to frequent panic attacks and bouts of depression. During her depressive and anxious episodes, Dee refused to go to school, she locked herself in her room, and turned to weed or cutting to self-soothe. She also experienced problems with sleep: she had difficulty falling asleep and stayed up late most nights.

Dee had seen a number of therapists before we began treatment, and she was hesitant to engage with yet another therapist. With Dee's complex presentation, I suspected there was something beneath the behaviors. During the assessment process, as she completed her Time Line activity, Dee shared that she had been sexually abused by an elderly uncle from the ages of 5 through 8. Dee was nonchalant as she shared this, but there was also a sense of detachment. I inquired about whether she had dealt with her history of abuse in previous treatment and she informed me that she was not believed. Her story of sexual abuse was seen as part of her lying/oppositional/attention-seeking pattern. Having her abuse validated and reported had a profound impact on Dee.

Initial treatment with Dee focused on safety and stabilization, and we had conjoint sessions with her mother to address feelings of anger and confusion Dee had about their relationship and her chaotic childhood. I met with Dee's mother a number of times as well to assist mother with regulating her own affect, to prepare her to hear Dee's thoughts and feelings, and to assist mother with attunement and interactive regulation skills. Dee readily engaged in somatic methods and expressive arts methods. We did a lot of work on boundaries and mindfulness (re: building blocks of experience), and these interventions improved Dee's self-awareness and capacity for self-regulation. Over time, Dee's relationship with her mother improved significantly, and Dee's functioning improved at school and in the home. She reconnected with interests and talents that had been neglected, and she developed a positive self-concept.

Table 6.1 The Many Ways Trauma May Present in Youth

Area(s) of Impairment in Youth's Functioning	*Frequent Diagnosis/Diagnoses (DSM-5)*
Anxious or fearful behaviors (including the need to recheck things such as doors locked, does not want to leave the home or go to school)	Generalized Anxiety Disorder, Obsessive Compulsive Disorder, Agoraphobia
Low mood, lethargy, lack of motivation	Depressive Disorder
Self-injurious behavior (including skin picking, hair pulling, head-banging, cutting)	Borderline Personality Disorder, Depressive Disorder, Trichotillomania, Excoriation, Obsessive Compulsive Disorder
Clingy, frequent crying or whining, regressive behaviors	Separation Anxiety, Reactive Attachment Disorder
Difficulty concentrating and focusing, memory problems, learning challenges	Attention Deficit Disorder, Learning Disorders, Intellectual Disability
Cannot sit still, high arousal, impulsive	Attention Deficit/Hyperactivity Disorder, Bipolar Disorder, Impulse Control Disorder
Frequent somatic complaints (e.g. headaches, stomachaches)	Somatoform Disorder
Use of alcohol or drugs	Substance-related and Addictive Disorders
Problems with elimination	Enuresis, Encopresis
Difficulty with social interactions, shy or withdrawn, inability to form connections with others	Social Anxiety, Autism Spectrum Disorder, Reactive Attachment Disorder
Eating-related concerns (e.g. binging, purging, food restriction, stealing/hiding food)	Eating Disorders, Hoarding Disorder, Kleptomania
Dislike of body, body-image issues	Body Dysmorphic Disorder, Gender Dysphoria
Inability to sleep or excessive sleep	Insomnia Disorder, Hypersomnia Disorder, Depressive Disorder
Bothered by intrusive thoughts, fears related to others watching	Psychotic Disorder, Schizophrenia
Does not respect rules or authority	Conduct Disorder, Oppositional Defiant Disorder
Rages, anger, aggression	Intermittent Explosive Disorder, Oppositional Defiant Disorder, Disruptive Mood Dysregulation Disorder, Conduct Disorder
Suicidality	Borderline Personality Disorder, Depressive Disorder, PTSD
Engages in frequent sexual activity with various partners	Borderline Personality Disorder
Frequently overwhelmed causing difficulties with breathing, and dsyregulation (physiological, emotional)	Panic Disorder

Part III

Somatic Interventions

Clinical Applications

7 Interactive Regulation

Because attachment needs are initially experienced and expressed primarily as body-based needs, the quality of the attachment relationship is originally founded on the caregiver's consistent and accurate attunement and response to the infant's body through their reciprocal sensorimotor interactions.

(Pat Ogden, 2006)

Ultimately, attachment relationships are all about how dyadic regulation shapes self-regulation. In other words, the child learns to regulate her own states of arousal and inner processing through interactions with another.

(Dan Siegel, 2012)

We begin our exploration of affect regulation with interactive regulation, also known as co-regulation, because interactive regulation is the foundation upon which the child's capacity to self-regulate is formed. Interactive regulation is the use of relationship to manage or maintain arousal within the window of tolerance. Interactive regulation can be a reciprocal process in that the caregiver is also impacted by the child's affect. Similarly, clinicians must be mindful of the bidirectional flow of affect regulation. Much has been written about the crucial role played by interactive regulation on the developing child's immature brain structures and nervous system (see, for example, Cozolino, 2006; Fisher, 2017; Schore, 2000; Sroufe, 2005). A child's first relationships are crucial to the development of neural networks involved in the capacity for self-regulation. The attunement of the attachment figure teaches the child, via neuronal activity, about safety in the world. Through attuned responses to the baby's cries, facial expressions, gestures, and movements, the caregiver provides interactive regulation.

In treatment with traumatized youth, we often encounter caregivers who are also dysregulated. There are myriad reasons for the caregiver's dysregulation, such as job or financial stressors, relationship conflict, and perhaps their own trauma history. Historical and other relevant information pertaining to possible family stressors is gathered during the comprehensive trauma assessment. The genogram can elucidate patterns of intergenerational trauma transmission. Moreover, research on epigenetics suggests that trauma effects can be genetically transmitted to offspring (Cozolino, 2006; Kellerman, 2013; Perry,

2014; Siegel, 2010 & 2012). Though in its infancy, epigenetics proposes that certain events, such as war, can alter genes and that the alterations are passed down through generations. For example, the grandchildren of survivors of the Holocaust or Canada's residential schools may carry, epigenetically, the trauma of their ancestors. Nijenhuis and colleagues (2010) propose that everything is epigenetic, or a combination of nature and nurture, such that the brain possesses potentialities that may be activated by experience. Thus, a child and family may come to us genetically predisposed and we must be prepared to work with both nature and nurture components. When this is the case, caregivers often require intervention to enhance their capacity to self-regulate. We can provide tools, through modeling and psychoeducation in the office, and suggest skill practice between sessions. Once caregivers are capable of monitoring and managing their own physiological states, they are in a better position to support their child.

Back to the Brain: Mirror Neurons, Polyvagal Theory, and Neuroplasticity

A few interpersonal neurobiological processes to keep in mind are mirror neurons, the Polyvagal Theory, and neuroplasticity. Moreover, we must remember that the human organism has an innate drive toward wholeness or healthy functioning, or organicity. Organicity is a foundational principle in both the SP framework and the Hakomi method (Johanson, 2009). Knowing that the human organism has an innate drive toward wholeness keeps us hopeful and motivated as we work with children and caregivers toward healing. Mirror neurons fire when the caregiver connects, through eye gaze, gestures, vocalizations, or facial expressions, with the child. Siegel (2010) refers to mirror neurons as the "root of empathy" (p. 29). Through the firing of mirror neurons, a synchronicity between affective experiences assures the child that her feelings, actions, and thoughts are real and that she is deserving of the affection and attention that she is receiving. In a way, mirror neurons enable an unspoken right-brain to right-brain (Schore, 2009) communication between the caregiver and child. Knowing, at an implicit or unconscious level, that the caregiver is fully present and accepting of the child engenders a positive sense of self and trust in others. Similarly, the caregiver and child mirror each other's affective states and movements in a way that is reassuring and affirming to the child.

Neuroplasticity, defined by Siegel (2007) as the mind's capacity to be altered by experience, offers opportunity for growth through therapeutic interaction and activity. Similarly, Doidge (2007) posits, in his seminal book *The Brain That Changes Itself*, that the brain is not a hard-wired machine as once believed, and that the brain's structure and function can be shaped or molded over the course of our lifetimes. Thus, regardless of the pruning (apoptosis) of under- or undeveloped brain structures or regions due to earlier experiences of neglect or abuse, the potential for growth exists. Porges' (2011) Polyvagal Theory identifies three distinct branches of the vagus nerve that play a role in affect regulation: the sympathetic branch, the dorsal branch of the parasympathetic system, and the newer myelinated ventral branch of the parasympathetic nervous system. Goldstein and Siegel (2013) note the utility of the evolutionarily newer myelinated branch, known as the social engagement system, in fostering growth when there is resonance with a trusted other. Therapeutic processes that involve dyadic interaction, whether between child and therapist, in groups, or in family work, have the potential to alter the traumatized child's dysregulated state.

Assess and Promote Attunement, and Enhance Caregiver Capacity to Self-Regulate

From the moment we meet the child and caregiver, we are assessing the quality of their interactions. Levine (2015) refers to a "basic discordance in their dyadic rhythm" that we can observe immediately. Does the caregiver respond with a soothing, prosodic tone? Do they offer physical comfort when the child is distressed? Do they mirror the child's state of excitement or joy in gestures, eye gaze, and tone of voice? Psychoeducation about the relationship between attunement and interactive regulation is important here, and it is essential that it be delivered in a supportive, non-blaming, nonjudgmental manner. There may have been traumatizing experiences that impeded formation of the attachment bond, such as the child witnessing violence between the caregivers or having been abused by the caregiver, or there may have been pre-birth or birth-related incidents that were traumatizing to the child and caregiver. Research shows that a secure attachment can be made with children despite the caregiver's own trauma history (Cozolino, 2006). We can facilitate connection through somatic methods more easily and quickly than with talk therapy, especially since most early memories are encoded on a body level as procedural memories.

A child's first relationships are crucial to the development of neural networks involved in the capacity for self-regulation. The attunement of the attachment figure teaches the child, via neuronal activity, about safety in the world. Through attunement to the baby's cries, gestures, movements, and silences, the caregiver provides interactive regulation. Babies learn to trust their own sensations by the caregiver's response. As noted in Chapter 2, the ARC framework manual offers a plethora of ideas for working with caregivers to provide co-regulation opportunities. ARC (2010) identifies two historical factors that contribute to the challenges of regulating affect with traumatized children:

1. attachment – the soothing interactive regulation with an attuned caregiver provides a foundation of positive experiences for the child to internalize;
2. traumatic stress response – due to exposure to overwhelming or chronic stress, the child does not develop a capacity to self-regulate.

When therapeutic settings, whether clinical, classroom, foster care, or residential treatment, and home settings consider these factors, there is greater likelihood that the child can get back on track with their developmental trajectory (Perry, 2006). Specifically, Perry states: "Healthy organization of neural networks depends upon the pattern, frequency and timing of key experiences during development." (p. 36). Bottom-up body-based approaches are most effective with traumatized youth given that the brain develops and changes in a use-dependent manner, and procedural (body-based) memories develop before episodic and declarative memories (Levine, 2015). Ogden and Minton (2000) note:

> Bottom-up processing…is initiated at the sensorimotor and emotional realms. These lower levels of processing are more fundamental, in terms of evolution, development and function: these capacities are found in earlier species and are already intact within earlier stages of human life. They precede thought and form a foundation for the higher modes of processing.

Through somatic interventions, we can model attunement as the caregiver observes our interactions with the child. We can teach caregivers to track their own and the child's responses to each other in various situations. Various activities give caregivers an opportunity to develop the skills of attunement (see Figure 7.1). Tracking, or monitoring, the building blocks of experience (5-sense perception, sensations, thoughts, emotions, movement) can provide a deeper awareness of the self, and of the self in relation to another. Steele and colleagues (2017) remind us that clinicians and clients are always communicating beyond the words, and the implicit messages elicit responses in each other. The ARC (2010) manual refers to the "parallel process" that occurs between child, caregiver(s), and clinicians when it comes to interactive regulation.

A distressed caregiver may be easily overwhelmed or triggered by their child's intense emotional and physiological states, and consequently they may be unable

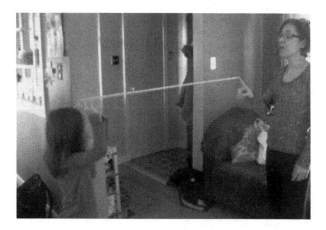

Figure 7.1 Attunement Activity. A mother and daughter navigate movement through a room, while remaining connected by their fingertips on a long wooden dowel, using only nonverbal communication

to attune to the child. The skills in Chapter 8 on self-regulation can be adapted and applied to work with the caregiver. For example, we can work with the caregiver's boundaries, proximity-seeking and avoidance, movements, and breath. Keeping in mind pacing; we work in a way that is tolerable yet expands the caregiver's window of tolerance. While the clinician may offer or create opportunities as an interactive neurobiological regulator (Fisher, 2017), there may be times when additional supports are necessary. Some caregivers are offered skill practice for use at home between sessions. Other caregivers may require referral to a group or individual therapist to focus on their own dysregulated affect.

Strategies to Promote Interactive Regulation between Caregiver and Child

Schore has written extensively about the process of "interactive psychobiological regulation" as occurs between therapist and client (Schore, 1999). As therapist, we are providing an experience of attunement for the caregiver, similar to that which is required between caregiver and child.

Movement and Body-Based Interactive Regulation Activities

Children and youth are more open to trying new things such as drumming or playing games. Their inherent inquisitive natures make somatic activities a great way to explore and enhance interactive regulation. As Perry emphasizes, there must be repetition in order to get a child back on their developmental trajectory (Perry, 2008, ch. 3). Specifically, he states: "Healthy organization of neural networks deepens upon the pattern, frequency and timing of key experiences during development." (Perry, 2008, p. 36). Bottom-up approaches are most effective, given the brain develops and changes in a use-dependent manner.

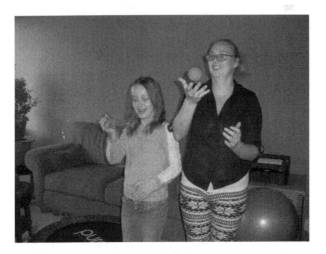

Figure 7.2 Mother and Daughter Play Ball in Interactive Regulation Activity

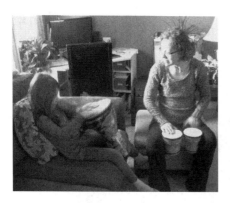 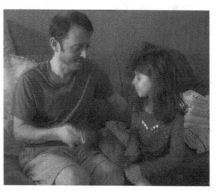

Figure 7.3 Interactive Regulation with
Caregivers Using Rhythm and
Musical Instruments

Figure 7.4 Interactive Regulation with
Caregivers Using Rhythm
and Musical Instruments

Singing (Porges, 2017), humming, and drumming with caregivers stimulate rhythm and offer opportunities for interactive regulation. Usually, I ask the child to lead and the caregiver to follow. Giving the child the lead gives them a sense of control and empowerment. It also gives us a glimpse into the caregiver's willingness to follow and ability to let the child do her own thing without correction or criticism.

Through curiosity and mindful experimentation, youth learn what type of input calms their nervous systems. In Figure 7.5, a boy is engaging in interactive proprioception activities. By developing an awareness of his inner experience and tracking his response to various inputs, he learned that he likes weight on his stomach while lying on his back. He experimented with lying on the physio ball and did not notice a shift in his inner experience; nor did he report a shift with the ball on his stomach alone. However, when the weighted dog was placed on the ball, his face lit up and he reported that it felt "good." We explored how he knew that from the inside, and he said

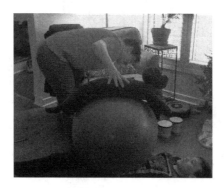

Figure 7.5 Interactive Proprioceptive Input

his stomach felt happy. Youth have different ways of describing their inner experiences. Since this youth was not a client, there was no preparation in terms of developing a somatic vocabulary or mindfulness of the inner experience. The shift that he noticed was evident on his face, however, and he was able to report something felt good for him. Children and caregivers readily engage in these experiments and they can easily be carried over into home practice.

As noted in Chapter 2, SMART (Warner et al., 2013) utilizes theory and technique from sensory integration, trauma theory, Sensorimotor Psychotherapy™, occupational therapy, and child development. The tools of the SMART room can be used for self-regulation and interactive regulation. With interactive regulation, the caregiver and child, or clinician and child, experiment with qualities such as rhythm, weight, movement, and proximity.

1. Small pop-up tent. Tents can be used for boundary work as well as self and interactive regulation. Children may want to go to the tent to calm or settle themselves, and the windows provide opportunity for co-regulation with caregivers or clinicians.
2. Djembe. This colorful drum tends to get children's attention quickly and they ask if they can play with it. In the office, stored out of view of this photo, are other musical instruments (maracas, tambourine, bongos, mini guitar) that can be used to facilitate interactive regulation.

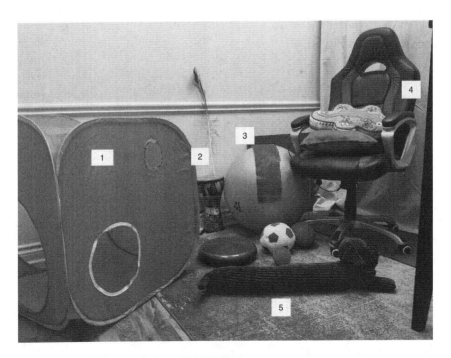

Figure 7.6 Regulation Tools for a SMART Room

3. Physio ball and physio band. The physio ball may be used for both interactive and self-regulation. For interactive regulation, the child may wish to sit on the ball to manage proximity to caregiver. Navigating distance through movement on the ball may enhance the child's capacities for both co- and self-regulation. Use of the physio band may help a child and caregiver explore and understand the connection between each other. For example, a child who has learned to use primarily self-regulation may develop the ability to tolerate a loose (limp band) connection to caregiver, in a way that does not feel intrusive or overwhelming. The loose connection with the band may then become a symbol of maintaining a connection with another in a way that feels safe and regulating.

4. Rolling/spinning chair. Some children crave vestibular input and a rolling, spinning chair may offer that needed stimulation. As with most of these activities, the child may choose to use it for self-regulation, but there are opportunities for co-regulation as well. For example, the caregiver can turn the chair at a speed desired by the child, or the caregiver might push/roll the chair. These movements are akin to rocking an infant.

5. Balls, cushions, and weighted objects. Balls may be used for rolling or tossing games for interactive regulation. Rhythm and repetition play a role in the enhancement of attunement and interactive regulation competencies. Weighted objects (the dog in this photo) and cushions provide opportunities for the child and caregiver to engage in interactive regulation via proprioceptive input. For example, the child may direct the caregiver as to what amount of weight and pressure feel better (see Figure 7.5). They can experiment with weight, pressure, and position on the body (e.g. belly vs. back). The wobble cushion (above the dog's tail in the photo) offers opportunities for interactive regulation. The child can stand on the cushion, balancing herself with the support of the caregiver. These dyadic dances, through repetition, foster trust in the process of interactive regulation.

    Note: There are other sensory tools, including a mini trampoline, behind the curtain.

> Dogs are not our whole lives, but they make our lives whole.
>
> (Roger Caras)

To close off this chapter, a final piece on interactive regulation and animals. Many of my young clients had a pet, mostly dogs, or they got an animal during the course of their treatment. Youth like Vincent and Dee were very attached to their dogs and often brought them to their sessions. The attunement and interactive regulation between them was palpable. There is a growing body of research on the neurophysiological benefits of human–dog interaction. A review of research by Odendaal and Meintjes (2003) found that positive effects in children include reduced cortisol levels, increased oxytocin and dopamine levels, lowered blood pressure and heart rate during pet presence, less aggression and more social integration, and improved mood. All of the aforementioned effects attest to the benefits of human–animal interactions. Levine (2008) writes about the ability to enhance the sense of groundedness through physical interaction with, or even simply observing the natural rhythms of, a cat or dog. Additionally, Beetz et al. (2012) found mutually beneficial results (e.g. increases in dopamine, oxytocin, and endorphins) from interaction between humans and dogs.

Case Illustrations

Dee

Dee and her mother attended the initial sessions together, and then I met with Dee separately. After a few individual sessions, it was obvious that Dee and her mother had very different views about their relationship. Dee's mother had shared her opinion that their relationship was close and she believed that her daughter confided in her. When together in session, Dee did not dispute her mother's view; however, Dee expressed anger about how her mother had "ruined" her life. It seemed that Dee felt she had nobody on her side, and she had felt unprotected growing up. In an effort to bring mother on board as a support for Dee, I invited her in for a session. Dee was made aware that her mother would be attending a meeting.

During the meeting with Dee's mother, it became apparent that there was a great deal of conflict at home and mother's reactions typically involved blowing up or detaching from her daughter. Dee's mother had a history of trauma as well, but we did not address her trauma in sessions. Instead, we explored ways that she could remain present and grounded when her daughter was explosive or defiant at home. We explored the signs of dysregulation in her daughter and developed ways to respond that were calming or, at the very least, did not escalate the situation. Through modeling and practice, Dee's mother learned how to use her body, eye contact, and prosody to meet her daughter's intense states. We also reviewed basic communication skills such as using "I" messages. For example, rather than raising her voice and moving her arms in an intimidating manner, Dee's mother agreed to try to speak softly, to give Dee space to express herself (safely, of course), and to position her body in a way that was less threatening. She also agreed to give space for Dee but to ensure Dee knew she was available when needed. After a couple of weeks, we had a joint session. Dee curled up tightly in the corner of the couch, covering herself with a cushion, as though she were trying to be smaller or invisible. Her mother sat at the opposite end of the couch, her body soft and relaxed into the cushions. Dee grew agitated quickly and her mother remained calm and quiet as she listened to Dee express her anger and resentment. Dee's mother's contained response was remarkable. After a minute or so, I moved my body and suggested through eye movement and prosody that mother offer a response to Dee. It was clear that Dee's mother was fighting off tears, but she managed to offer reassuring words. An exchange ensued during which Dee could be seen settling, her voice calmer and clearer, her body relaxing, and she was able to make eye contact with her mother. We had another joint session a couple of months later: Dee's mother appeared more attuned and Dee was more receptive and communicative with her mother.

Adele

Adele shared that she had recently resumed cutting herself with a razor blade. I reminded her of the limits of confidentiality that were covered when treatment began, and I asked her how she would like to proceed with creating a safety plan. Adele was only 13 and her cognitive functions were lower than her chronological age so it was important that her caregivers be involved in the safety planning. Adele was reluctant to include her caregivers in the planning. We explored Adele's reluctance and she indicated that her father was always away for work, and she felt that her mother's reactions were too much. She thought her mother could not handle her strong feelings of sadness and hopelessness. Adele's mother presented as stoic. Since the caregivers were not present, we agreed to call Adele's mother to discuss a safety plan. During the phone call, Adele said very little. She appeared nervous and mostly nodded or shook her head in response. Through prosody with mother on the phone and gestures with Adele in the room, we were able to bring them together to develop a transparent safety plan. I validated mother's strong feelings and fear for her daughter, while reminding her that her daughter needed her to be present by using a steady, firm, yet gentle voice. The safety planning resulted in the cessation of self-injurious behavior, but Adele and her mother never did develop close, trusting communication.

Vincent

When in the office with his mother, Vincent presented differently than during individual sessions. I noted his lengthened spine, minimal shaking and fidgeting, and his gaze tended to rest on his mother's face. Vincent appeared to be containing himself while in the presence of his mother, who tended toward a hyperaroused state when discussing Vincent's trauma history. Vincent's mother was aware that we had been working on ways for Vincent to feel safer and manage his physiological state. She was understandably concerned that Vincent might return to self-injury or substances to cope with his overwhelming PTSD symptoms (e.g. nightmares, flashbacks, hypervigilance, depression, and isolation). However, it was clear that Vincent's mother was incapable of co-regulating him.

I suggested we engage in an experiment using the emwave. Vincent had used it previously during an individual session and he liked how it slowed his breathing down. He actually purchased one for practice at home and he tracked his progress by connecting the device to his laptop. With curiosity, I wondered if they would take turns with the emwave. Since Vincent had used it before, he knew how to operate the device so he set his up, hooked his mother up, and provided instructions. After five minutes, Vincent's mother was unable to establish coherence with the emwave feedback, so Vincent gently asked if he could try. Within a minute, Vincent established coherence and the unit's lights and beepers went off. His mother was intrigued and asked how she could do that, so I suggested that she come in for a meeting to discuss affect regulation. She agreed, and we met twice.

During our meetings, I provided information about the process of interactive regulation and shared my observations about the difference in Vincent's presentation when she was in the room. Vincent's mother broke down in tears, sharing her feelings of guilt for having not protected her son, the heartache she experiences whenever she sees him in distress, and the helplessness she feels about the systems of care that they were involved with. His mother was also traumatized by her son's abuse (secondary traumatization) and required some assistance to get regulated. She was an extrovert, energetic woman who gesticulated a lot when she spoke, which she attributed to her culture. Through grounding, breathwork, and centering, she was able to provide a calming, regulating presence for her son.

8 Self-Regulation

As the child's brain matures into the preschool years, the emergence of increasingly intricate layers of self-regulation becomes possible.

(Dan Siegel, 2015)

Recent trauma research highlights the relationship between childhood abuse, other adversities such as neglect and poor attachment with a primary caregiver, and impaired self-regulation. Some youth may exhibit high arousal (hyperarousal), and others might present with extremely low arousal (hypoarousal). Additionally, some youth may vacillate between the extremes, presenting at one moment as hypervigilant and the next as avoidant or shut-down (Cloitre et al., 2009). Impaired self-regulation can negatively impact functioning in many domains (see Figure 8.1). As van der Kolk (2008) asserts, affect regulation is the most important intervention in therapy and, as discussed in Chapter 4, a felt sense of safety (internal and external) is critical from the beginning of treatment. Some youth want to dive right into the water (process their trauma); thus it is our responsibility to educate them about needing to be resourced (able to self-regulate) first. As my EMDR trainer Barbara Horne said, you can't climb Mount Kilimanjaro with just a granola bar and flip-flops. Children of all ages get this. We can begin by ensuring that the child feels safe in our office setting and then explore the ways they know this from a somatic perspective (e.g. what in your body tells you that you're safe?), model self-regulation, and use somatic interventions to facilitate the capacity to self-regulate and feel safe internally. This chapter identifies the ways complex trauma may manifest across domains, provides information about sensorimotor processes related to affect regulation, and offers strategies to help bring young clients back into a place of optimal functioning.

Optimal Arousal or Being "in the Zone"

Every child has his own optimal arousal zone. In other words, what is slightly beyond manageable for one child might be perfectly tolerable for another child, while another child might be overwhelmed. Dan Siegel (1999) described

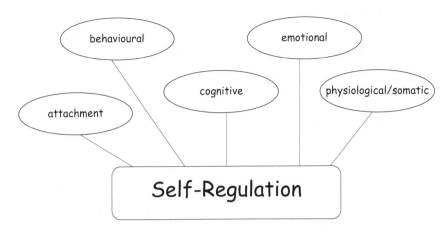

Figure 8.1 The Key Areas Impacted by Dysregulated Affect in Traumatized Youth

these zones and coined the term "Window of Tolerance" (WOT). Other descriptors of the same concept include Pat Ogden's "modulation model," Sandra Wieland's "window of receptivity," and Peter Levine's "window of self-regulation." In treatment, I encourage young clients to find the words that make sense for them. Since our clients are all unique, we need to spend time exploring what feels overwhelming, or underwhelming, and what feels tolerable for each individual. In my practice, youth have used different names for their optimal arousal zone, including "When I'm okay," "center," "just right," "happy place," "calm zone," and "in the zone." See Figure 8.3 for the beginning of one youth's window of tolerance (WOT). Over time, the youth adds to each zone the effects on cognition, emotions, sensations, and actions/movement (see Figures 8.6 and 8.7 for an example of a youth's completed WOT later in this chapter).

One of the first steps in helping youth recognize where they are vis-à-vis the WOT is to teach them to track their inner or somatic experiences. We may need to teach them the difference between feelings (emotions) and what we feel inside (physical sensation). Some youth, especially younger children, have limited vocabulary and benefit from creation of their own lists. Ogden and Fisher (2015) call this a "somatic menu." The menu is often created on a white board with younger children because they enjoy the process of writing (and drawing) on the board themselves. If the list is created on a white board, we may have to erase it when the session ends, so we might copy it onto a sheet of paper or take a photo (caregivers often take a picture of the list for future reference). Teens have taken their lists and carried them in their pockets or backpacks for practice between sessions. See sample somatic menu below.

Sample Somatic Menu

heavy	jumpy	bright	jagged
dense	fuzzy	pale	rubbery
hot	still	cool	bumpy
cold	swirly	warm	smooth
tingly	prickly	silky	popcorn
ticklish	tight	rough	hollow
empty	open	sandy	shallow
full	closed	loose	deep
sharp	bubbly	fluffy	butterflies
wavy	dense	soft	sticky

Working with the "Window of Tolerance"*

High arousal (hyperarousal) – fight/flight/flight responses manifest as panic, impulsivity, hypervigilence, rage, racing thoughts, body tension, feel unsafe, emotional overwhelm

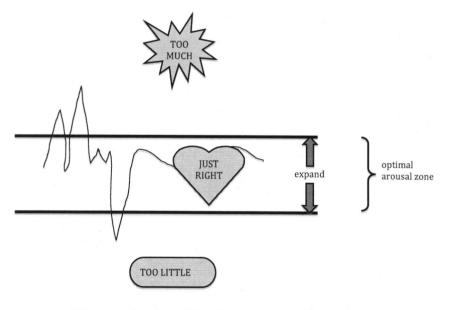

Low arousal (hypoarousal) – collapse/feigned death response manifests as numbness, slowed movement, slowed thoughts, no energy, shut down, hopelessness, disconnected, shame

Figure 8.2 Child-Friendly Adaptation of the Modulation Model

Source: Ogden, P. & Minton, K. (2000). Modulation Model [Image]. Sensorimotor Psychotherapy: One Method for Processing Traumatic Memory. In *Traumatology*, Vol. VI, 3(3), 1–20.

* Window of Tolerance. Siegel, D. (1999). The Developing Mind. New York: Guilford Press.

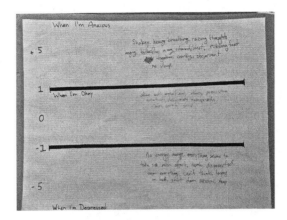

Figure 8.3 Youth's Creation of Arousal Zones or Window of Tolerance

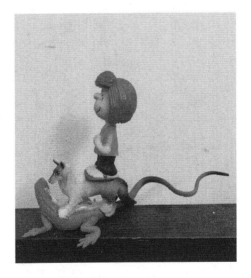

Figure 8.4 Triune Brain Model for Children

Ways to Help Youth Know When They Are Within or Outside Their Windows

Body Feelings Map (BFM)

As with most components of therapy, whether during assessment or treatment, psychoeducation is useful. Use brain models or explanations of the mind–body connection to help clients understand the purpose for engaging in activities. Tailor psychoeducation to the client's age and developmental stage. With younger children, I use a child-friendly model of the triune brain that I created (see Figure 8.4) to illustrate the connections between the three brain levels (brain stem, limbic, cortex), and to explain the need for collaboration between the three levels if we want to manage intense emotions and sensations. Somatic and creative activities can be used to assist in the exploration of what feels right and what is "too much" or "too little." We can be playful and model curiosity with interventions. An initial activity used, as part of my assessment process with all clients, is the Body Feelings Map (BFM). I first learned about this activity from the supervisor (Debbie Dukes) of a children's mental health program where I worked in South Carolina, and I have modified the process through experience with youth over the years. Depending on the age of the child, a one-page coloring activity can illuminate his experience of a range of emotions. The activity provides useful information about his emotional awareness, how he experiences feelings on a somatic level, how he expresses feelings to others, and the sources or triggers for his feelings. With younger children, a full-body outline and a lengthier process are used. I preface this activity as a way to help us both understand what happens inside and outside when we have feelings, and explain that we work from the inside out. Depending on the child's self-awareness and ability to articulate, this activity can take two to three sessions. The main components of the BFM are:

1. Introduction – Introduce the activity and draw the outline.
2. Color – Invite the youth to indicate where they notice feelings inside their body using colors.
3. Inner experience – Once coloring is complete, explain that we cannot see what is happening on the inside and invite them to describe for you. If not already done, provide or create a somatic menu and prompt for somatic (sensations) descriptors.
4. External expression – Invite the youth to describe how they show each of these emotions to others.
5. Sources (or triggers) – Usually a between-session task, the youth is asked to journal/identify three sources of each of the feelings.

Next, we shall describe the main components of the BFM in detail.

1. Introduction

The therapist draws a human figure outline, sort of like a ginger bread person. Use humour to model capacity to tolerate imperfection with artistic endeavors, especially with youth who might be reluctant to engage in this task due to perceived lack of artistic ability. Draw the outline using the color that they had previously identified as their favorite, a demonstration that you have been paying attention to them from the beginning.

2. Color

Hand the image to the client, on a clipboard for support, along with pencil crayons. Explain that we are exploring how feelings live in the body, or how feelings are experienced inside. Choose words that match your style and the client's developmental stage. Let them know that pencil crayons are used because they allow us to see overlapping colors more easily than other mediums such as markers, and that they may discover that several feelings live in the same place. Some children will ask why we use pencil crayons because they have a preference for markers, pastels, etc.

Ask the child to refrain from talking while coloring their feelings. Explain that we are using different parts of the brain than those involved with speaking and thinking. Some children cannot refrain from talking while coloring and that is fine, too. Remember we are meeting the client where they are and following the client's lead when possible. With youth, we can elaborate our explanation with right-brain (creative, emotional) and left-brain differentiation. For those that require a more concrete description, I use 3-D wooden mannequin and brain models to guide exploration and enhance understanding (see Figure 8.5 for an example). Inform them that you are asking them to color feelings that most people experience at some time in their lives and they can choose whatever colors they want for each. Suggest they create a legend so we can remember what each color represents. Also, reassure them that some feelings come more easily than others and they might want to close their eyes (or soften their gaze/look ahead on the floor for those not comfortable closing their eyes) while they recall a time that they felt that way. This may help them sense what lights up inside with that feeling.

The set of emotions asked about are: sad, jealous, angry, guilty, scared, anxious (younger children seem to understand worry better than anxious), and happy. After happy, I invite them to add any other feelings they have sometimes, suggesting that they could add that feeling with a color not yet used. Adolescents, more than children, like to add a couple of other emotions (e.g. bored, confused, shame).

3. Inner Experience

Once the coloring is complete, explain that you want to understand what is going on inside for them. If you have not yet done so, provide them with a somatic menu (see above) or invite them to create a menu of their own. You can prompt them with simple sensations such as buzzy, hot, cold, heavy, etc.

4. External Expression

Next, I ask the youth how they share their feelings with others, or how I might know they are feeling something (e.g. sad). Younger children and youth from non-demonstrative families might struggle with this piece. With younger children, I might bring out a mirror, so they can look at themselves to learn how

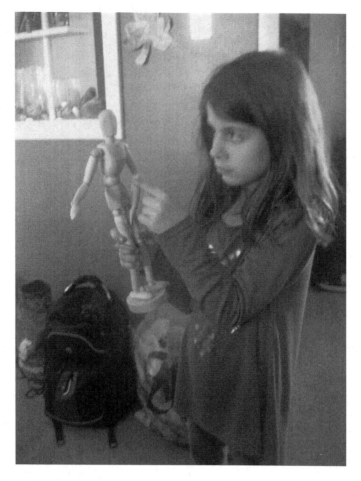

Figure 8.5 A Child Uses a Wooden Mannequin to Identify and Express her Somatic
          Experiences

they express feelings. This can be a fun piece of the BFM. For others, I might
ask them to find images in magazines that reflect each of the feelings. A few
words about non-demonstrative families. There may be factors contributing
to lack of emotional expression that require clinical intervention; however,
we need to be mindful that some cultures have a tendency either not to show
their emotions, or there are some emotions where expression is more acceptable than others. When clinical intervention is indicated, I have brought in
the family for games, such as feelings charades, to facilitate recognition and
expression of emotions in service of the youth. Feeling word charades involves
family members forming teams, pulling a card with a feeling word or face, and
demonstrating through facial expressions only. Again, this can be a fun activity,
and it can also be diagnostic.

5. Sources

The final component of the BFM is completed between sessions. Youth are invited to select a journal to do this piece. Children of all ages enjoy receiving something to take home. We must be sure to include journals that appeal to all ages. These are usually purchased at low cost, such as dollar store items. After the BFM has been copied (color copy) or the youth has taken a photo (everyone has a smartphone these days), invite the youth to write the following:

> Three things that make me feel sad, jealous, angry, guilty, scared, anxious, happy (and whatever feeling the client added to the list).

Explain that it can be anything they have felt in the past or present. This explanation is given because some clients think they are being asked to write what they feel between sessions. I often give the example, "For happy, I would write puppies, ice cream, and my motorcycle." We want them to have choice so inform them that they can use images or draw the sources rather than write. Assure them that it is okay if they cannot come up with three for each.

A final note about the BFM. Children with histories of neglect, trauma, or abuse often lacked the ability to engage in mobilizing (fight/flight) defenses during the abuse. Subsequently, freeze or collapse may be more familiar responses. The truncation of the mobilizing actions may appear in the BFM. For example, the child may have no color on his legs or arms. The BFM is completed at the beginning of treatment because it offers diagnostic information that informs treatment interventions.

Children's Windows of Tolerance (or Zones)

Another activity that explores children's awareness of their capacity for self-regulation is the creation of their own window of tolerance (WOT). This can be done on a piece of construction paper or large flip-chart paper. Younger children gravitate toward the larger surface because they can draw and add stickers to their zones. Depending on the age and developmental level of the child, a caregiver may be present to help identify indicators. For example, younger children often have difficulty knowing and naming what they do to calm themselves. Sometimes I offer a chart to assist the youth and caregiver (see Figure 8.6) with this activity. As listed in the chart, we help the youth identify their cognitive, emotional, somatic, and behavior functioning within each of the zones. The chart is laminated so that the child and caregiver can review and circle their experiences.

By the time we begin working on the youth's personal WOT, we have a sense of their functioning in each of the zones. For example, the youth may have been referred due to self-injurious behaviors such as head-banging or cutting. We may not, however, know whether these maladaptive attempts to self-regulate stem from feeling too little or too much. We can explore this with them, asking what is happening inside and energy-wise when they self-injure. It is also

Table 8.1 Zones of Regulation

	Thoughts	Feelings	Actions	Sensations
Hyperarousal (too much)	• Racing thoughts • Concrete/inflexible • Rumination • Disorganized or hyperverbal language • Difficulty formulating clear thoughts • Disconnected from reality	• Anxious • Angry • Hypervigilant, on edge • Lack of emotional attunement	• Little eye contact • Lots of movement • Impulsive • Disjointed movements • Lacks body awareness	If able to connect to the body and report: • Electricity • Popcorn • Tension • Vibrating • Tingling • Hot or cold
Best possible arousal (just right)	• Coherent thoughts and language • Flexible thinking • Oriented to time/place/situation (per developmental stage)	• Able to feel and express range of emotions • Can feel connection to others and experience attunement	• Integrated/controlled movements • Body awareness and able to reach for/meet basic needs • Synchronicity between movement level and heart rate/breath	If able to connect to the body, and depends on age/developmental stage: • Connection • Calm • Relaxed • Lightness
Hypoarousal (too little)	• Impoverished thoughts and language • Disconnected from reality • Limited orientation to time/place/situation	• Low energy and little motivation • Feels numb or dead • Limited or blunted Affect • Hopelessness	• Sluggish or slow movements • Collapsed	If able to connect to the body and report: • Heavy • Slow • Pressure

possible that self-injury is used in states of hyper- and hypoarousal. As the youth is completing his zones chart, we are exploring the adaptive function as well. For example, perhaps running up and down the hallways at school prevented him from recalling painful memories of his stepfather beating his mother. Or, wetting the bed at night helped stave off the sexual abuse she endured as a child. We want to help clients recognize and accept that some unconscious actions (fight/flight/freeze) were helpful in the past but may no longer serve a purpose. Again, we are providing psychoeducation throughout treatment.

Children and youth can be taught activities and skills to self-regulate. Self-regulation is essential to managing internal states and external behaviors, whether in the classroom or at home. As noted in the previous chapter, the capacity for self-regulation is developed though the interactive regulation with the primary attachment figure. In neglectful or abusive households, children often do not receive this critical developmental piece. Once a variety of strategies have been learned, they can be added to the back of the client's personal WOT. Clients write five or six strategies on small pieces of paper and slip them into the back pockets after the page has been laminated. A summary of steps for the personal WOT:

1. Draw and name the zones (three sections as illustrated in Figure 8.6).
2. Identify the impact of too much, too little, and just right, on cognitive processes, emotions, actions/behaviors such as sleep patterns, movement styles, and sensations. Once identified, they are written, drawn, or otherwise placed within the zones. Younger children enjoy adding stickers to their creations.
3. Create pockets for the back of the page and mark them accordingly (see Figure 8.7). The page is then laminated before the next step.
4. Assist the youth to select strategies that have already been identified as effective at down and up-regulating and write them on small pieces of paper. The paper slips are placed into the pockets and the window is ready for the youth to take home.

Hyperarousal

Hyperarousal has received more attention than hypoarousal in the research and literature because the behaviors exhibited by hyperaroused youth are more noticeable and troubling to others. These behaviors tend to be externalized, such as aggression, impulsivity, and defiance. Overt signs of hyperarousal might include:

- fast, pressured, or tangential speech;
- frenetic energy and constant movement; disorganized movements;
- irritability, easily angered, or easily overwhelmed; panic attacks;
- lack of eye contact (could be many reasons for this but something to notice);
- impulsivity;
- body tension;
- more subtle signs – rapid or shallow breathing, cold/clammy/pale skin.

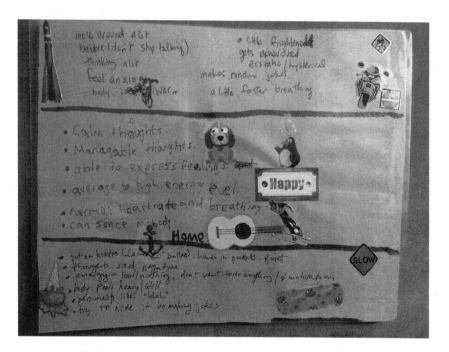

Figure 8.6 Youth's Zones (or Customized Window of Tolerance) with Pockets on the
Back to Hold Regulation Activities/Techniques

What we may not readily observe: racing thoughts, sensitivity to rejection,
obsessive thinking or rumination, internal sensations that accompany high
activation (e.g. tingling, vibrating), and disconnection from reality.

Activities to Down-Regulate

Choice of activity is geared to the client's strengths and interests. Psychoeducation,
in language that makes sense to the individual developmental level of the child,
is offered to help them understand how these activities might benefit them.
Anytime the youth engages in a novel activity, something that is non-habitual,
there is opportunity to settle the nervous system and expand the window of
tolerance. Often it is a matter of bringing them back to their bodies through
these activities, thereby getting them out of the fight/flight/freeze response.

1. grounding;
2. alignment;
3. balloon breathing/abdominal breathing/smell the flower–blow out the
   candles (or blow the pinwheel)/hiss;
4. bounce while sitting on a physio ball;
5. orienting to present space and time;
6. weighted blanket/pillow/stuffed toy;

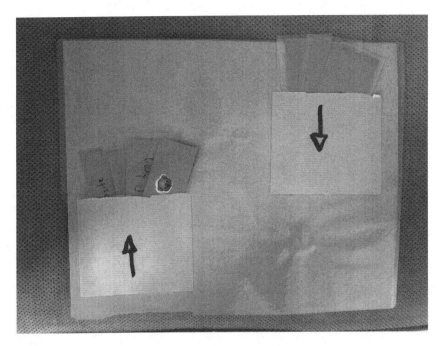

Figure 8.7 Youth's Zones (or Customized Window of Tolerance) with Pockets on the Back to Hold Regulation Activities/Techniques

7. rhythmic movements like shooting hoops, walking slowly (mindfully);
8. qigong/tai chi/yoga movements.

Grounding is essentially bringing awareness to your feet on the ground, sensing the stability of the ground beneath you. This can take the youth's attention away from the racing thoughts and calm agitation in the body. With younger children, I usually make grounding activities playful, such as inviting them to imagine their feet are in muck and they are pushing through the muck to the solid, dry ground beneath. We can be playful with talk of squishy muck between toes, etc., in the service of getting their attention on their feet connected to the solid ground. We might expand the imagery to the feet having roots that go down into the earth and connect to others. With older children and youth, simply asking them to notice their feet on the ground, move them front to back/heel to toe, and from side edge to side edge, sensing the contact with the floor, is sufficient. Another activity children and youth like for grounding is coloring mandalas. The act of coloring, without worry about going outside the lines of circular images, is grounding in itself. I keep a variety of mandalas in the office to introduce the idea and, if youth are interested, they may download images off the internet or purchase them at bookstores/dollar stores.

Alignment involves lengthening the spine, which allows youth to breathe into areas they might not usually. From a somatic therapy approach, alignment and grounding are two of the first techniques used for safety and stabilization (Gene-Cos et al., 2016). Fight/flight/freeze responses typically create short, shallow breathing, and alignment enables the breath to become more expansive, fuller in the body. Youth have also reported that they feel stronger, more empowered, through grounding and alignment. See Chapter 10 for alignment activities.

There are myriad breathing activities that we can introduce and experiment with in sessions. Breathing also crosses over into other areas such as qigong movements and yoga poses (detailed in Chapter 10). Colleagues have talked about using square breathing with clients, but I prefer a rectangular breathing structure because the image suggests a longer exhale. I might use an index card, which the child can decorate as she chooses, to practice this breathing method. Relaxation happens on the exhalation so we want to teach our clients to breathe out longer, even if only one second longer. During this, and all activities listed throughout this chapter, we are checking in with our clients to notice shifts (e.g. "What changes, if anything, when you breathe like that? Does your breath get slower, or fuller? Let's just notice what happens when we breathe like that"). We are also slowing them down as they bring their awareness to the breath, calming the sympathetic activation. Balloon breathing, usually used with younger children, might go something like this:

> Let's put one hand on our bellies and one hand on our chest and breathe normally. Notice which hand is moving more? (Most children will say the top hand is moving more.) Ok, now let's imagine that we have a balloon in our bellies. It's a blue (or their favorite color) balloon. Now we are going to breathe in through our noses, aaalllll the way down to fill that balloon with air. Let's try together. (Therapist demonstrates the technique, making sure that the lower hand on the belly moves out with the inhalation, while observing the child's ability to breathe into her belly. Children often do not get this the first time so I suggest different ways they can practice.) Ah, that's good. I wonder if there is a way to make the balloon get fuller. Hmmmm, sometimes it helps to lie down and put something on the stomach, like a pillow or stuffed toy. Want to try? (Be sure your client is comfortable with lying on the floor as some children do not feel safe doing so. If that is the case, we can suggest they try at home instead.) Once they have achieved the ability to make the toy or pillow move with their breathing, they are quite pleased with their accomplishments and eager to demonstrate for the caregiver. At the end of the session, we may invite the caregiver in to observe the child's newly mastered skill.

Hypoarousal

Children experiencing hypoarousal are often overlooked due to their quiet, withdrawn presence. They may seem sad at times, or morose as teens. Subtle signs of hypoarousal in youth include collapsed shoulders and body, slowed or no movement, and the appearance of being spaced out. Note that a medical (e.g. slow movement in muscular dystrophy) or cognitive impairment (e.g.

impoverished speech in alogia or traumatic brain injuries) must have been ruled out as causal factors. Other signs of hypoarousal:

- flat affect;
- low energy, lethargic;
- impoverished speech;
- detached;
- low/no motivation;
- hopelessness/despair/sadness;
- appearance of daydreaming or spaced/tuned out;
- flaccid or limp musculature.

Signs of hypoarousal are more difficult to detect given they are usually the absence of something, such as numbing, connection, impaired cognitive processing, or emotional expression. In some children a few of the above symptoms may be more pronounced, while there may be a combination of symptoms in others. As clinicians, more time and attention may be required to track and notice the signs of hypoarousal, especially if they are inconsistent. For example, the youth may have a different presentation with and without the caregiver(s) present.

Activities to Up-Regulate

1. stand, movement (e.g. walk, wave arms over head or side to side);
2. breathing into the upper chest;
3. jump on mini trampoline;
4. hum, sing, chant;
5. activate the ventral vagus (through social engagement, e.g. therapist uses prosody and eye contact; or, splash or touch face with cold water);
6. tapping the legs, or butterfly hug;
7. bouncing, kicking, tossing, or rolling a ball back and forth;
8. qigong movements.

Children with complex trauma histories often experience PTSD as well as co-morbid depression. If we are able to help them find something they were/ are interested in and strengthen that interest, we can bolster their essential resilience (remember the principle of organicity). While writing this section, I pondered the healing power of music in traumatized youth, reflecting on the numbers of youth who either constantly pumped in tunes through earbuds or became engaged in learning an instrument as part of their healing process.

Nightmares and Flashbacks

Youth often "relive" their trauma through intrusive images in the form of nightmares and flashbacks. Since they do not usually know the triggers, we want to help them identify triggers through sensory activities. Teaching them to be mindful or more aware of their physiological state in present moment experiences enhances their ability to identify triggers. Rothschild's (2000) protocols are an excellent tool to help young clients manage flashbacks and nightmares. We review them together in session, and then clients take them home for practice/use. Clients are reminded that it is beneficial to practice the protocols when not needed, as with most strategies, so they can come to them quickly in times of need.

Nightmare Protocol

If I wake up after a nightmare feeling _____, and notice
                                  (name a feeling, usually scared)

_____ *in my body* because I just had a bad *dream* about
(notice what is happening in your body)

_____, I will *look around* where
(name the nightmare, no details)

I am *now* in _____ in my _____.
              (this year)   (name room, e.g. bedroom at home)

As I look around and see _____,_____,_____,
                              (name three things you see right now in this room)

I will know that I am awake and safe and that the nightmare is not happening anymore.

Adapted with permission from Babette Rothschild's protocols in *The Body Remembers: The Psychophysiology of Trauma and Trauma Treatment*. New York: W. W. Norton, pp. 133–134.

Flashback Protocol

Right now I am *feeling* _____,
                    (name a feeling, usually scared or fear)

and *sense* _____, _____,
(describe what is happening in your body, name at least two things)

because I am *remembering* _____.
                    (name the trauma by title only, no details)

I am looking around where I am *now* in _____ here in my _____.
                                        (this year)   (place you are now)

and I can see _____, _____, _____,
                    (name three things you see right *now* in *this room/place*)

so I know that _____ is not happening anymore and I am safe.
          (name the trauma by title only, no details)

Adapted with permission from Babette Rothschild's protocols in *The Body Remembers: The Psychophysiology of Trauma and Trauma Treatment*. New York: W. W. Norton, pp. 133–134.

Vestibular and Proprioceptive Systems

Two sensory systems impacted by neglect and traumas are the vestibular and proprioceptive systems. As Teicher et al. (2003) posit, severe early neglect and maltreatment "produces a cascade of neurobiological events that have the potential to cause enduring changes in brain development" (p. 33). These children have great difficulty with focus and attention; thus learning is a challenge. Spinazzolla (2016) notes that these children "can't attend to school based learning because most of them are attending to more important learning, survival, based on what happens when I go home tonight" (J. Spinazzola, JRI [Justice Resource Institute] presentation, July 29, 2016, via YouTube). Development of these systems in infants requires movement and attunement from the caregiver (Warner et al., 2012). Children with underdeveloped vestibular systems may have difficulties with sensory processing, coordination, movement, and balance (Doidge, 2015). We might observe these children constantly seeking stimulation (e.g. spinning in chairs, rocking back and forth, and jumping or bouncing movements). The vestibular system, part of the inner ear structure, involves balance, awareness of self in space, and position of our heads. Simply put, proprioception involves input from muscles and joints through touch. Warner and colleagues (2011) note: "Proprioception moves the individual to an organized state from a place of high or low arousal, beautifully providing up-regulation or down-regulation depending on the need of the organism." (p. 20). Neuroplasticity promotes development or rewiring of these systems through activities that youth can engage in within the clinical setting.

We will observe our young clients automatically gravitate toward the activity that meets their needs. For example, I worked with an 8-year-old girl who spent the first 40 minutes of our initial sessions bouncing on a Pilates ball. During the first two sessions, I noticed that she could not sit still on the sofa, either getting up to move and returning to the sofa frequently or fidgeting constantly, and she stuttered at times. Part way through the second session, I invited her to sit on the Pilates/physio ball instead of the sofa. She loved it, bouncing constantly for the remainder of that session, and she immediately sat on the ball upon arrival to subsequent sessions. Over time, her stuttering disappeared, the time on the ball decreased, and the speed of bouncing slowed. When they arrive, many of my youth (and adults!) either remove their shoes to knead the textured wobble cushions, or they grab the weighted dog that sits on the back of the sofa. Still others hold a pillow on their laps or play with a crocheted unicorn sitting on the sofa. Finally, I learned about a method for proprioceptive input from an OT colleague (Ellen Yack, personal communication): creation of a personalized tapping tool. The client is assisted in the process of creating a soft, weighted tapping tool using a couple of socks filled with rice. Through demonstration, she is taught to tap her arms with the tool in a rhythmic way with the amount of pressure that feels right for her. Typically there are five taps on the back of the hand, five taps on the forearm, and five taps on the upper arm (outside of the bicep area). The customized tapping tool seems to be something youth continue to use on their own over the course of treatment, and some youth have

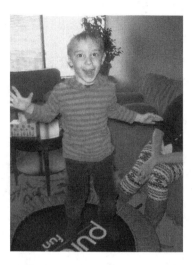

Figure 8.8 Vestibular and Proprioceptive Input

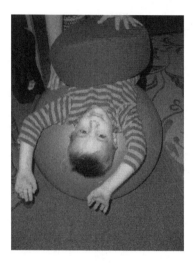

Figure 8.9 Vestibular and Proprioceptive Input

gone on to make their own weighted blankets. This activity can also provide a sense of containment. In Figures 8.8 and 8.9 there are photos of children engaging in vestibular and proprioceptive activities.

Brain Gym

Brain Gym is a movement-based method used to enhance learning ability. Brain Gym, developed by Paul and Gail Dennison (1992), is based on the principles of kinesiology and involves bilateral stimulation. In 2009, I attended an introductory workshop, led by Paul Hyman, and I have been using the PACE activity with clients ever since.

P Positive (hook-ups)
A Active (cross crawl)
C Clear (brain buttons)
E Energetic (sip water)

It is done in reverse order, starting with E.

While Brain Gym was developed as an educational tool to improve capacities such as focus, attention, and memory for students, it can also induce calmness in children. A series of four movements that goes by the acronym PACE can be useful at the beginning of a session, to settle and bring the client more present into the room, during a session, to enhance integration, or at the end of a session to provide a calming container. There is much research that suggests crossing the midline, or bilateral stimulation, facilitates bilateral integration of the brain (e.g. Goddard-Blythe, 2011; EMDR). Many descriptions of PACE are available on the internet. Here are basic instructions for PACE:

1. Drink water (Energetic)
    Dehydration diminishes cognitive capacities so taking a drink of water is like oiling the machine (machine = brain).
2. Brain buttons (Clear)
    Place one hand across your upper chest slightly below the collarbone. With the thumb in one indentation and the index finger in the other, press lightly on these points for approximately 30 to 60 seconds.
    Place the other hand over the navel or belly button.
    For younger children, a butterfly hug can substitute for this move.
3. Cross crawl (Active)
    While standing, reach the right hand across the body so that the hand touches the left knee as you raise it, and then do the same with the left hand to the right knee. For more of a challenge to those with great flexibility, connect the elbows to the knees instead. Do 15–20 of these movements.
4. Cook's hookup (Positive)
    While seated, cross the legs at the ankles. Next, reach the arms forward and cross the hands over at the wrist so they clasp. Lastly, in a downward motion, bring the clasped hands under and then up until they are resting on your chest.

Breath

Breathwork is touched upon in Chapter 10 but we shall cover a few additional strategies here. A child can be overwhelmed when there are too many external stimuli. In these times, it is helpful to shift their orientation to their internal self via breath. For example, we might ask him to simply notice where his breath is, how deeply it is moving, whether it is fast or slow, and whether the breath feels

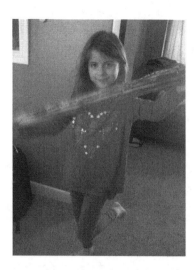

Figure 8.10 Rainstick Breathing

smooth or trembly. When there is too much happening on the inside (e.g. child feels anxious and is experiencing racing thoughts, rapid heart rate), we might direct her attention to the external environment. For example, we might ask her to find something blue or a round object in the room, and check in about any shifts in breath. Youth can be taught to track shifts in their breath simply by changing their awareness between inner and outer experience. Youth can also gain a sense of empowerment when taught to pendulate (Levine, 2008) between the pleasant and unpleasant experiences.

Youth can be taught to breathe into different areas of their bodies to activate, or calm, the nervous system. If a boy appears collapsed, lethargic, detached, or numb, he may be in a state of hypoarousal. Sometimes the collapse is a truncated flight response, so inviting him to stand is a simple way to activate him; however, he may not wish to accept our invitation to stand at this moment. Alternatively, we might suggest that he try breathing into his upper chest, modeling the breath as we make the suggestion. Upper chest breathing activates the sympathetic and social engagement systems (remember Polyvagal Theory). For those in a hyperaroused or a highly activated state, we want to slow down and shift the breath into the abdomen, through diaphragmatic or belly breathing, to activate the parasympathetic (rest and digest) system.

Centering

Grounding and centering can have similar effects but are not quite the same. Centering is bringing our awareness to our midline or our core. Ogden & Fisher's (2015) Hand on Heart/Hand on Belly is an exercise I frequently use with youth. It offers a tangible way for young clients to connect somatically to their core or center. We can center to calm ourselves through strategies such as focused breath or imagery. Youth respond well to imagery connected with breath. For example, we might ask them to imagine a streaming light, like a pillar or column of light, moving in through the core with each inhalation and exiting through their feet with the exhalation. Increased centering can occur if we ask them to imagine, then contact with their hand, the horizontal middle of the body simultaneously. Centering is particularly useful for states of hyperarousal. Qigong and yoga movements can be centering as well.

Tools to Concretize Self-Regulation Skills for Youth

Coping Skills Toolboxes

One activity many youth enjoy is creating their own coping skills toolkits or toolboxes. The kits can be made from a shoebox or any kind of container. Contents depend on the individual child as they are creating a kit of ways to regulate based on needs. Some youth decorate their boxes and this can be regulating in itself, and provides opportunities to enhance social engagement as they are freer to talk when focused on an activity that they enjoy. Prior to the use of SP in my clinical work, I explored affect regulation with youth through the five senses, but SP has enriched my understanding and, therefore, the range of areas to include. Core organizers, or the building blocks of experience, are now integrated into the toolkits. Over the past few years, I have been creative in finding ways to individualize and concretize youths' skill sets. Completed kits typically contain visual, tactile, olfactory, auditory, and gustatory items that provide a sense of calm (or whatever sense the youth names as helpful to regulate, such as happy box or centering kit). There are also reminders of movements, places, or people that settle them back into their windows of tolerance. The youth take their kits home once complete.

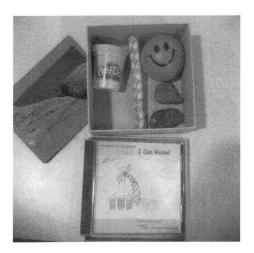

Figure 8.11 Coping Skills Toolboxes

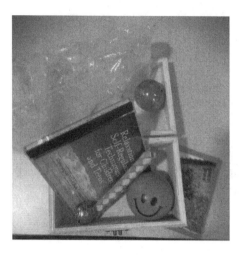

Figure 8.12 Coping Skills Toolboxes

From SP: 5-STEMS

Acronyms are a great mnemonic device for teaching and help youth remember. I created '5-stems' to help youth learn and remember the building blocks of present moment experience (Ogden & Fisher, 2015). Through fostering curiosity and engaging in experiments, youth discover what makes them feel better or calms their system (or activates, for those living in hypoarousal). I offer small wooden cubes for youth to decorate as a reminder of the 5-stems (see Figure 8.13). Additionally, youth create a cube, based on a generic cube for illustration purposes (see Figure 8.14), that identifies the sensory stimuli and a movement that they have discovered brings them back into the window of tolerance. Most youth come up with names for their cubes, such as calming cube or happy dice, depending on the purpose. Youths' completed cubes might include fabric, scented oils, or magazine photos of images that reflect the sounds, tastes, sights, scents, and tactile sources that benefit them. We find ways the cube might help each client, such as rolling it and engaging in whatever activity turns up (e.g. take a walk in the park – movement; pet the dog – touch; take a lavender bubble bath – touch, scent). One client asked to take his box home before it was finished, because he liked the idea of rolling the dice and following through with the designated sensory activity.

Tools to Demonstrate Flow of Emotions and Sensations, and Foster Sense of Control

Another concrete tool that exemplifies a sense of control over somatic (and emotional) experience is taps (faucets) that the client can actually turn. The visual and tactile connection is a tangible way for young clients to "get" that they can turn it

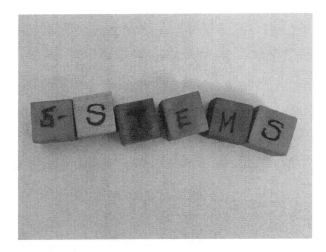

Figure 8.13 Wooden Cubes to Represent the Building Blocks of Experience (5-STEMS)

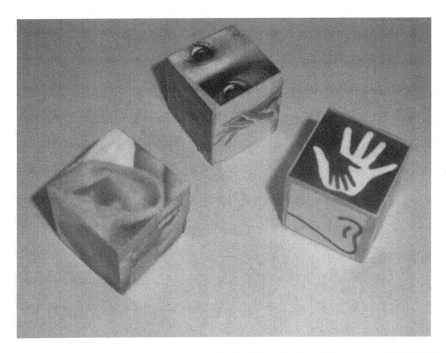

Figure 8.14 Wooden Cubes to Represent the Building Blocks of Experience (5-STEMS)

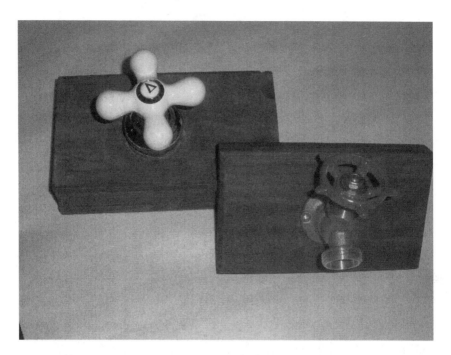

Figure 8.15 Concrete Symbol of Capacity to Turn Emotions Up/Down or On/Off

up or down, on or off. I have created tools for use in the office (see Figure 8.15) for children to experiment with and, if this is something that helps them regulate, caregivers may go out and purchase a similar tap/faucet combination from their hardware or plumbing store. The tool can be included in the child's toolkit.

One client expanded on the tap/faucet concept. Dee, mentioned in other chapters, was creative and artistic, and she found that creative activities facilitated her healing process. After we talked about the symbol and she experimented with turning the tap, an image came to her and she asked if she could paint it. As Dee created a watercolor painting of a water fall, she frequently closed her eyes and tuned into her inner experience. Dee felt safe being in nature, with the sounds and smells surrounding her, and she made a beautiful painting of this creative resource. On the top of the waterfall, Dee painted a large, faint faucet to reflect connection to the activity that sparked the image.

The Emwave

The Emwave is a portable feedback device developed by the HearthMath Institute. Youth can install software that enables them to play games and receive coaching through their Emwave connection. The Emwave measures heart rate variability (HRV), the variability between one heart beat and the next. High HRV levels reflect low stress levels. As van der Kolk (2014) notes:

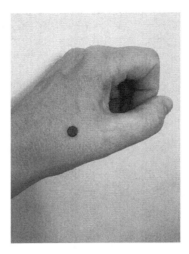

Figure 8.16 Biodot on Hand

"HRV can be used to test the flexibility of the system, and good HRV – the more fluctuation, the better – is a sign that the brake and accelerator in your arousal system are both functioning properly and in balance." (p. 77). Porges (2011) has written extensively about the role of the vagal brake, or the myelinated vagus, in affect regulation.

Biodots®

Biodots are tiny skin thermometers that can be worn on the child's hand throughout the session. These little dots, like the mood rings from decades ago, change color based on the child's skin temperature. The best location for the Biodot® is the area between the thumb and index finger (see Figure 8.16). Like a portable biofeedback device, the child can get a sense of when there is too much tension and practice their calming techniques. Additional information about Biodots® is listed in the appendices.

See Table 8.2 for a summary of regulatory activities. Note that some techniques appear in both columns because they can be useful depending on the individual and the situation. It can be a matter of bringing the child back to the present moment, out of the fight/flight/freeze/collapse response. As we get to know our young clients, and through mindful experimentation, we can help them build a repertoire of skills.

Containment

We all have a natural container – our body is our container. Activities can help youth get a sense of their edges and this may aid in increasing their tolerance for strong emotions and sensations. Remember to teach clients the difference

Table 8.2 Regulatory Activities Summary Chart

UP REGULATE	DOWN REGULATE
Stand, walk	Balloon breathing/belly breathing/slow, deep breaths
Balloon badminton	Weighted blanket/stuffed toy
Kick, toss, or roll ball back and forth	Bounce on Pilates ball
Drumming or other percussion instrument	Smell the flower, blow out the candles/pinwheel
Brain Gym	Drink water through a long straw
Breathe into upper chest	Qigong, tai chi, yoga
Yoga – warrior pose	Focus on breath
Rub hands together (stimulates contact, warmth, energy) – consider adding hypoallergenic, scent-free lotion, depending on client and her trauma	Orienting to present time/space
Engage the five senses (e.g. Dolan's orienting exercise)	Grounding
Tap legs/arms	Alignment
Humming	
Alignment	

between avoiding or repressing feelings/sensations and containing them. A container allows clients to feel a sense of control over overwhelming sensations, feelings, thoughts until a time when they might feel more able (i.e. safe, stable) to tolerate and manage the intense sensations and emotions. Some clients experience a sense of containment by wrapping a blanket around themselves. Some younger children get a sense of containment from being surrounded by body socks (Ellen Yack, personal communication). Body socks, used by occupational therapists, are composed of stretchy fabric. They can be purchased or made from material found at fabric stores. Techniques from Sensorimotor Psychotherapy™ (Ogden, Minton & Pain, 2006; Ogden, 2015) and Somatic Experiencing® (Levine, 2008 and 2013) help us to become aware of our container – the body:

1. Self-hug container (Peter Levine – NICABM, 2013 Trauma Therapy Webinar Series): Place one hand under the opposite armpit, then the other hand over the other upper arm (bicep region). As you settle in this position, notice your breath, any tension, and other body sensations. Sit with this as long as you can and notice any shifts in thoughts about self, other, and the world.
2. Push against the wall or doorway: feel the container created by your arms, the wall, and your shoulders/back. Check that knees are slightly bent and then push into the wall, sensing the strength and the circular energy within your arms, shoulder/back, and the wall. Try pushing from your core, again noticing the circular, contained energy arising.
3. Visualization of container (includes sensations/5-sense perception).

Container visualization is used in many treatment models and frameworks, including EMDR and Sensorimotor Psychotherapy™. While I have been using this intervention for many years, my method has expanded through my training in these models (SP, EMDR). Children and youth with the capacity to visualize find this intervention helpful and they appreciate that they can engage in the activity to bring about containment in any setting (e.g. on a bus, in the classroom). Following is an example of a script I might use to guide a youth through the process of visualizing a container.

- Take a moment to settle into the chair (or sofa). Notice the support of the floor under your feet, the chair supporting your back, and take a few slow, easy breaths.
- When you're ready, imagine a container that will hold all your worries and fears. This container will allow you to leave the upsetting thoughts and feelings behind so you can go on with your day when you leave here. You will be able to return to these worries and fears later, but for now we will put them away.
- Get a sense of the size and shape of your container. *(pause)* Now, notice the color and texture of your container. *(pause)* Okay, next, imagine a lid or top that closes and locks. *(pause)*
- Now I'd like you to imagine putting all your worries, fears, distressing feelings and thoughts into the container. *(notice if the child appears puzzled or confused and offer something concrete such as: imagine you are folding them up like pieces of paper or soft cloth)* Place them gently into the container. These are your thoughts and feelings and we need to be gentle with them.
- Once you have placed all your worries, fears, thoughts, and feelings into the container, imagine you are closing the lid of the container. Close the lid and make sure it's locked. Know that you can return to these thoughts and feelings when you are ready but for now we are going to put them away.
- Now, imagine that you are putting the container somewhere safe, maybe on a shelf or under the stairs. Take a moment to find just the right place for your container. *(pause)* When you are ready, walk away from the container and return to the room.

Note that wording is individualized based on the youth's developmental level and presenting concerns. For example, worries and fears might be replaced with anxieties, or angry thoughts, or scary feelings.

4. <u>Tapping legs/arms</u>: Tapping along the arms or legs provides a sense of containment as it increases awareness of one's edges and reconnects to the body. Youth can do this with their hands or an object. Some youth prefer to use objects such as stress balls or they create their own tapping ball,

while others simply tap with their hands. Younger children find it regulating when their caregiver does the tapping for them (i.e. interactive regulation). The interactive regulation also provides opportunities for the child to notice what feels right, in terms of speed and pressure, and to communicate this to their caregiver. Levine (2008) provides detailed instructions for safety and containment tapping exercises that can easily be adapted for use with youth.

Case illustrations

LGBT+ group

Based on clients' expressed interest and need, I created and offered a group for LGBTQ+ youth. The somatic-based group was similar in content to a group I had developed previously for adolescent girls who had been sexually abused. This group, however, was specifically for LGBTQ+ youth who had body image issues and a degree of phobia of inner experience related to their sexual orientation, internalized homophobia, and shame regarding their histories of sexual abuse. All of the youth had expressed a wish to be in a group of other LGBTQ+ youth and I was not able to find one in the city so I created one. I was fortunate to have an SP student, Sonny Berenson, a trans-identified man, to co-facilitate this group.

The group focused on experimenting, in mindfulness, with somatic experiences to enhance their self-awareness and the capacity for self-regulation. They engaged in various activities, including proprioceptive or vestibular input, containment, breathwork, and pendulation, and then they recorded their responses on a sensory record (see below). Group members came together to discuss their experiences, and they also shared other creative resources with one another. Being in this group with peers, and the witnessing of each other's experiences, were validating, normalizing, and regulating. This was not a research project, however, and youth's completed pre- and post-tests (e.g. CPSS – Child PTSD Symptom Scale, 7–17 years) reflected improvements in a number of areas including mood. Afterward, in individual sessions, youth reported that the group was a positive experience for them and that they particularly appreciated the opportunity to engage in the somatic experiments in the presence of their peers. This sharing was huge given many of these youth were introverted and had difficulty in social situations.

Additional Illustration

Vincent often turned to art as part of his healing process. He found that he was able to express himself through art in ways that he could not otherwise.

Table 8.3 Tracking Form

Building Block	Touch	Taste	Sound	Smell	Sight
5-Sense Perception					
Sensation(s) & Location(s)					
Feeling(s)					
Thought(s)					

Like Vincent, musicians may find healing in their writing and music-making. I reached out to a friend about her healing journey through music. Following is an excerpt from an interview with this singer/songwriter:

> My childhood trauma happened in the house. I lived on a farm and we were very secluded, so I couldn't escape. My parents had mental health issues and it was a bit of a roller coaster. On the outside I appeared happy, outgoing, friendly and social, but my inner world was a little sad. I escaped the confusion and sadness by turning to music...I got a guitar in my teens, locked myself in my room, and put my feelings to music. I learned how to make my own music, to write and play. Writing my feelings into songs, it was like a connection to a higher power. I grew up in a religious family and was connected to faith, and I felt loved, like answers came to me in my music. It was not a thought process...comes from heart, soul and body.
> The skill of learning and playing – it took a lot of time learning the skill of playing and singing at the same time.
> Something happens physically, it's a vibrational thing, like the body is on fire. I had put a lot of walls up, blinders on, pretending everything was fine but I was in pain. An early song I wrote was Stop, Look and Listen, a song to a mother about a child that was unlovable. Other early songs were called, Fuck You, Will You Comfort Me? (about suicide, asking God when will you be there for me), and Am I Annoying You?

The depth of the adolescent's inner turmoil and pain are reflected in her early song titles and lyrics; moreover, her innate resilience led her to reach for a way to express herself in learning to play guitar and write her own music. This young woman found healing power in her musical refuge.

9 Boundaries, Proximity-Seeking, and Avoidant Behaviors

> Traumatised children are often easily dysregulated by relational dynamics, and often experience the sequential or simultaneous stimulation of defensive and proximity-seeking impulses toward their caregivers.
>
> (Pat Ogden, 2015)

Infants are born pre-programmed to seek proximity to their caregivers for their very survival. The developmental movements (yield, reach, grasp, pull, and push) used by babies facilitate and maintain the connection to a primary attachment figure. Over time, the caregiver's response, or lack thereof, creates a pattern of expectations to proximity-seeking behaviors (Ogden, Goldstein & Fisher, 2012; Ogden & Fisher, 2015). Consistent, responsive, attuned caregiving forms the foundation for the development of the child's capacity to reach out in times of distress. As Schore (2003) notes, prolonged periods of distress, through caregiver's rejection or harsh response to baby's distress, can be toxic to the infant's rapidly developing mind and body. Ultimately, the child develops internal working models (IWMs) about the self and others, and these IWMs impact their sense of safety and trust in relationships. The child's ability to form healthy boundaries may be compromised to the detriment of developing skills required to form social relationships, learning, and self-esteem, which, in turn, may lead to victimization or chronic health issues later in life.

Internal Working Models (IWMs)

Bowlby's (1973) attachment theory proposed that infants develop internal working models (IWM) from birth, based on the patterns of early interaction between the infant and primary caregiver. According to Bowlby (1973), "each individual builds working models of the world and of himself in it, with the aid of which he perceives events, forecasts the future, and constructs his plans" (p. 203). Thus, an individual's IWM contains perceptions about the self, others, and the world in general, and creates predictions about what to expect from people and situations. As Ogden (2014) notes: "Procedural learning reflects internal working models." (p. 91). Children that experience responsive, receptive caregiving learn that their wants and needs, and indeed their very existence, are good. However, if the child's caregiver is not attuned and efforts to have needs met are thwarted or rejected, they may develop a negative IWM. A negative IWM may engender a sense of inadequacy or a view of the self as bad or unlovable. With a negative self-concept, children are less likely to seek social interaction, assistance in a learning environment, and comfort and support when distressed.

When distressed, a child with positive IWMs may seek support when threatened, such as if being bullied during recess in the school yard. As Pietromonaco & Feldman Burnett (2000) write, individual's IWMs are most likely to be activated when threat is perceived, leading the child to reach out for support from a trusted other. However, if the child has not learned to trust others will be there for them, they may engage in self-destructive or aggressive behaviors in efforts to fend off the perceived threat. The child's IWM and default defense responses are activated at a subcortical level, and the consequences typically confirm the IWM of self as bad, unworthy, or unlovable.

Faulty Neuroception

To summarize, neuroception (Porges, 2017) is the autonomic nervous system's unconscious evaluation of environmental cues regarding safety. When working well, children can respond appropriately to protect themselves or reach out for support when needed. As Ogden and Fisher (2015) elaborate, "the neuroception of safety is reflected in the inhibition of defense systems and in activation of behavioral flexibility that enables adaptive contact with others: reaching out, grasping, eye contact, holding on, letting go, pulling toward, pushing away" (p. 30). To function in school, family, and community settings, children require behavioral flexibility. To illustrate, play is a healthy activity for children and play frequently takes place within school and community settings. Indeed, Panksepp's research identified a brain system implicated in play (see, for example, Panksepp, 2010; Badenoch, n.d.). Early trauma and attachment experiences with rejecting, critical, or frightening caregivers can impede children's capacity to play (Ogden & Fisher, 2015). Play can be rough, as in wrestling or a game of football with friends, and thus children need to accurately assess threat and safety in order to engage in these play activities without activating the sympathetic nervous system's fight or flight response.

As advanced by Porges' Polyvagal Theory, we have a social engagement system (ventral parasympathetic branch of the vagus/tenth cranial nerve) that promotes interaction with others and the environment (Ogden, 2015; Ogden & Fisher, 2015; Porges, 2017). According to Porges (2017), "if we lose the capacity of this newer vagal circuit to regulate physiological state, we become a defensive fight/flight machine." (p. 66). Children with complex trauma and attachment injury often have compromised social engagement systems. As van der Kolk (2014) notes, a great deal of energy is required to continue functioning with reminders of trauma and the resultant feelings of terror, shame, and vulnerability. One can easily imagine the challenges a traumatized child faces in forming relationships with peers when they are depleted through constant dysregulated states and relevant neurological systems are inaccessible.

Let's turn to an illustration of faulty neuroception in the life of a child. Suppose a child grows up in a home with interpersonal violence involving frequent yelling and loud sounds, for example. We would expect his sympathetic nervous system may be highly sensitized, he may be in a state of constant hyperarousal, and he may be hypervigilant. Below consciousness, this child may be activated by the slightest sensorial reminder and react as though he is in danger. Loud voices may be triggering, resulting in the neuroception of danger. To return to the football reference, if the child is playing football and someone yells across the field or runs quickly toward him, the child might be triggered into a fight or flight response. The faulty neuroception of threat can lead to disastrous consequences in social milieus, such as ostracizing or physical assault by peers, further entrenching the child's negative view of self. Subsequently, they may isolate and avoid social interactions altogether, no longer reaching out for connection, or the efforts to be in relationship could be misdirected with aggressive, controlling behavior.

Social Engagement

Just as humans are wired for play, humans are also wired for social engagement. As noted above, Porges (2017) has identified a newer myelinated branch of the vagus nerve specifically related to social engagement. Additionally, Schore (in Stein & Kendall, 2003, p. 191) writes about the impact of a rejecting caregiver, meant to serve as an interactive regulator as the child's prefrontal cortex develops, on the biochemistry of the brain contributing to subsequent problems with social behavior and impulse control. Finally, Perry (2011) laments about the changes in current society that limit the connections children have with others, and the deleterious effect on the development of children's regulatory capacities.

Social engagement increasingly takes place through social media, and children spend countless hours communicating with others or playing games with their smartphones and video game systems. Though this field is in its infancy, research results about the impact of social media on youth's social skills and social engagement are mixed (see, for example, Steiner-Adair, 2013). Caregivers, too, may be preoccupied with their email and social media, modeling relational disconnection and reducing the opportunity for interaction necessary to stimulate growth in brain regions implicated in social engagement. We may observe the impact of intergenerational transmission of trauma in the gravitation toward social media interactions as caregivers with their own trauma histories may lack the ability to balance closeness and distance (Ogden, 2015).

So how does the lack of development of social engagement processes affect proximity-seeking and avoidant behaviors? Children and youth may be more inclined to turn to more anonymous supports through their online communities. Additionally, the time spent in online interaction takes away from face-to-face relational opportunities. Youth may become self-reliant in the sense that they do not see the point in reaching for support or connecting to others beyond the screen. Communicating behind a screen cannot develop the social engagement muscles that Porges (2017) writes about. Ogden & Fisher (2015) define social engagement as "a set of circuits including the ventral vagal nerve that stimulates engagement with the environment and other human beings through our facial muscles, eye movements, voicebox, and turning and tilting of the head" (p. 776). This input is lost behind a computer/phone screen. Youth who are sensitive to criticism and have fears of rejection may have a preference for onscreen social interaction. Unfortunately, the number of youth with experiences of cyberbullying is rising. A Canadian study found that nearly one in five internet users between the ages of 15 and 29 were victims of cyberbullying or cyberstalking (StatsCan Canada, 2016). An exploration of this topic is beyond the scope of this book. As a therapist, encouragement of face-to-face social interaction may become a treatment priority with some youth.

Boundaries

Messages about boundaries are primarily communicated nonverbally through gesture, posture, movement, and facial expressions. Sensorimotor Psychotherapy™ emphasizes psychoeducation about boundaries and somatic experiments with boundaries, especially in phase one treatment. Ogden (2012) specifies two types of boundaries to work with in treatment (physical and process), and identifies three functions of boundaries: containment, screening, and protection. A physical boundary refers to space, proximity, and distance. Process boundaries are the individual's internal processes including thoughts and emotions. The three boundary functions may appear different across contexts. The containment function can be viewed as a filter or choice in what the child shares with others or keeps to herself. For example, she may wish to fully express her emotions with her family or with close friends, but opt to contain (e.g. dampen or limit) emotional expression in her school setting. Screening is about what to allow in and what to keep out. Fay (2017) describes the use of boundaries as a way to tolerate differences, to recognize what is their opinion or value versus someone else's. We can see how ineffective boundaries may come into play, especially during adolescence where identity formation in a social context is critical, leading to difficulty with decision-making and vulnerability to negative peer influences. Ogden (2015) notes that the need for proximity in relationship, as well as needs for distance and boundaries, are innate to humans. She elaborates that "relational trauma can disrupt this dyadic dance of intimacy and boundaries between children and caregivers" (p. 139).

How do boundaries develop? Scaer (2007) writes that "we receive positive or negative information as a developing infant or child from sensory experiences that contribute to our unconscious perception of safe boundaries" (p. 3). Repeated negative messages might, over time, instill the belief in a child that he does not deserve to set limits or boundaries, or that the wants and needs of another (i.e. the caregiver) are more important than his. He may eventually suppress all wants and needs, perhaps even develop a view that children who express wants and needs are weak. The natural give and take that is required in social interaction may be impeded by the erection of impermeable boundaries. Fay (2017) suggests that the individual's attachment style contributes to tendencies to either distance from, or merge with, others. The child who received negative messages about his needs, such as dismissal or humiliation, leans toward a distancing measure. On the other hand, the need to merge or enmesh (no boundaries) may occur when a child has experienced caregiver neglect or inconsistent messaging. Individuals with a tendency to merge boundaries, not know how to set boundaries, or that it is even possible to do so, can have far-reaching effects in childhood as well as later intimate relationships. Relational trauma is a boundary violation (Ogden & Fisher, 2015). Most youth with histories of complex trauma are unable to set flexible, adaptable boundaries.

Now, let us consider some common scenarios before we move to interventions for working with boundaries and proximity-seeking/avoidant behaviors. Imagine for a moment the child who:

> Followed behind his mother to hide the razor blades she used to cut her wrists; the child who gathered the beer bottle empties after her father passed out drunk, hoping he would stay asleep and she could get some rest without worrying about him coming to her room at night; the hungry 4 year old who looks at his bruised, crying mother, eventually developing the ability to ignore body signs of hunger and, ultimately, suppress all needs; the 10 year old who has learned to stand up for himself, get what he wants at any cost because his father taught him that is what a man does and his mother humiliated him when he expressed the need for comfort as a little boy. How might the development of proximity-seeking and boundaries be impacted by the experiences of these youth? What limiting beliefs about self and others may be internalized, impeding the abilities to form healthy physical and internal boundaries?

Clinical Interventions for Working with Boundaries, and Proximity-Seeking and Avoidance

Working with Proximity-Seeking and Avoidance

Proximity-seeking behavior is inherently regulating (Bowlby, in Stein & Kendall, 2003). Working with movement while fostering curiosity and play can expand children's capacity to reach and connect. We can design somatic experiments for children and their caregivers, working with the developmental movements, for example, to facilitate proximity-seeking behaviors. As Ogden and colleagues (2012) note: "Children may develop an implicit prediction that no one will respond to proximity-seeking behavior, and thus literally abandon integrated, purposeful proximity-seeking actions. In therapy, helping children to become more aware of their procedural tendencies and practicing new actions can address these types of issues." (p. 12).

Experiments are done in mindfulness at a slowed pace to enable youth to attend to the moment-by-moment unfolding of their experiences. The slower pace in itself may challenge habitual patterns and, as noted in Chapter 2, we want to facilitate an experience that is different from patterned responses in order to create growth. As Cloitre (2015) asserts, one-size-fits-all approaches to trauma treatment are inadequate and we, as clinicians working with traumatized youth, need to remain creative and attuned as we strive to meet the needs of individual youth and families. Following are activities that help traumatized youth to explore and develop proximity-seeking behaviors:

- Pilates band, piece of rope, or towel: invite the youth to reach as you extend the item to them. Ask for a report in mindfulness. Note: mindfulness reports are made as present-tense statements. For example, "I feel tension in my arm and want to pull away." Some clients may find it difficult to reach, and we can modify the activity so that we are facing away or our gaze is averted from the youth. Especially for youth triggered by perceptions of vulnerability, we can alleviate the concomitant sense of shame by not watching as they engage in the reaching action. Some youth may want to quickly grab the extended item (habituated response to stay in proximity with caregiver), so we encourage them to slow down, using soft prosody and assurance that we are here. We then ask them what it is like to hold the item. Once they give a report of the impact on building blocks (sensations, etc.), we may tug gently and ask them to notice what happens when we tug. We might also invite them to tug gently and notice what that is like for them (pulling toward). Again, the range of responses depends on the beliefs youth have about being in connection with another person. Some youth will smile and say it feels good. Finally, explore what it is like for them when you, the therapist, drop the other end. This can be provocative in youth that desperately crave proximity, but it can offer a sense of relief for those who do not feel comfortable with connection. One young person stated that they felt sad when I let go of my end, immediately followed by feelings of disgust for "acting like a baby." It is important that we have an understanding of the youth's attachment style, capacity to track or monitor their own experience, and that they have tools to help them return to their windows of tolerance before we begin these experiments.
- Distance – movement away and toward. Using a rolling chair or large physio ball, invite the youth to notice what happens when you move away from them. Ask them to get a sense of what distance feels right for them. What impulses, sensations, thoughts, and feeling arise as you create distance between the two of you? We can also reverse this and invite the youth to engage in the movement. Remember, these are experiments and there are no wrong ideas; just model curiosity as you check out the experience

of creating distance for the youth. If there are impulses, we can invite the youth to follow through with the impulse. For example, they might want to reach out as you back away, or they may feel an impulse to tilt their head and smile as you move closer. The latter may be a signal that the youth is beckoning you to come closer.

A reminder about the need to reframe traumatized youth's avoidant strategies, such as isolation, aggression toward self or other, or dissociation, as survival strategies. Help the youth recognize that a strategy that was helpful growing up in an abusive household was adaptive at the time but may no longer be useful in their current situation. Also, maladaptive proximity-seeking behaviors, such as sexualization or somatization (i.e. an attach cry), may have served a purpose when they were in the abusive or neglectful environment. The child learned what she had to do to stay in proximity with an abusive caregiver. Framing maladaptive strategies as survival skills helps alleviate the sense of shame and guilt children may feel. Ogden (2014) notes that, "over time, infants will learn to repeat the expressions, postures, movements and gestures that elicit a desired response from their attachment figures, or, at least in traumatogenic environments, minimize abuse and neglect" (p. 90). The gestures, expressions, postures, and movements become procedural tendencies that operate below client awareness. This piece of information is also important to share with youth as it helps mitigate the shame and blame they may feel about their behaviors.

Working with Boundaries

Clinical interventions that address boundaries with traumatized youth may be the youth's first experience of having an adult respect their boundaries. The ability to recognize and assert a boundary is crucial to a child's sense of safety and agency. A child living with a depressed caregiver, for example, may prioritize meeting his caregiver's needs at the expense of his own. He may internalize implicit or explicit messages that he is selfish and bad if he refuses to comply with his caregiver's request. Subsequently, the youth may find it difficult to set limits and boundaries in relation to others, or he may develop beliefs that he is unworthy and his needs do not matter. We can engage youth and caregivers in exploration of boundaries, both physical and internal (process), and facilitate the development of flexible, adaptable boundaries.

- Creation of a physical boundary (e.g. with yarn/string/pillows). An example of a tangible boundary appears in Figure 9.1. The young girl pictured played with sitting and then standing in the giant, flexible sphere. Her favorite part was that she could stand up and still feel surrounded by something. In practice, youth with complex trauma histories have gotten into the sphere and curled their bodies inward. Experiments progressed through reaching out with eye contact, then movement beyond the edge of the boundary (e.g. putting a finger, hand, then an arm through an opening).

The clients study the experience, through the building blocks (e.g. sensation, impulse, feelings, thoughts, and 5-sense perception), of reaching toward another, then retreating back to safety. These experiments give them a sense of having a boundary in place while remaining in relationship with another. Playfulness, for those comfortable with play, and mindful curiosity are features of boundary experiments.

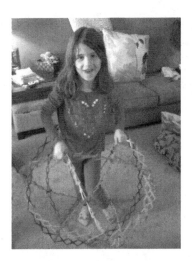

Figure 9.1 Young Girl Experiments with Creation of a Boundary Using Giant, Flexible Sphere

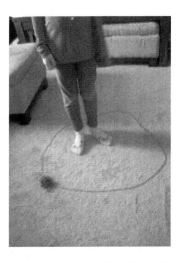

Figure 9.2 A Girl Experiments with Getting the Right Size and Dimensions for Her Boundary

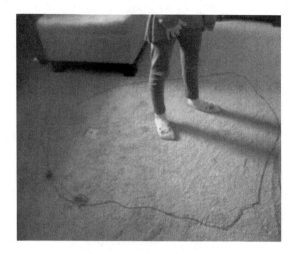

Figure 9.3 A Girl Experiments with Getting the Right Size and Dimensions for Her
        Boundary

- Negotiating boundaries – for self, and with another. In Figures 9.2 and 9.3,
  an 8-year-old girl experiments with creating a boundary from yarn. After
  exploring how it felt inside the boundary, and how her body told her it was
  "just right," she enlarged the boundary. She stated that it felt like she could
  not move with the smaller boundary, and she did not like the "feeling" of
  not being able to move. The "feeling" was experienced as overall rigidity
  and tension in her body, and a sense of being stuck in place as though her
  feet were glued to the floor. Once she expanded her boundary, the girl
  shared that she felt lighter, freer, and she liked that there was room for her
  to invite someone in if she wanted.

The next image (Figure 9.4) presents siblings negotiating boundaries. The
older sibling expressed frustration that her younger brother was always getting
into her things and into her space. Her younger brother was very affectionate
and seemed to lack awareness of personal space. The children recognized that
their boundaries with each other might be different from boundaries with
others, such as friends, teachers, or their caregivers. Remember that these
youth are not clients and they possessed a sophisticated self-awareness that
is not typically seen in clinical practice with traumatized youth. The siblings
experimented with different boundary sizes and shapes until they got just the
right boundary for their relationship. They also explored and practiced ways
to express their needs for closeness and distance with each other.

I am reminded of an adolescent that I worked with a few years ago. Mother
was very protective of her daughter as her daughter had a long history of school
and social problems related to severe affect dysregulation. The adolescent was
prone to aggression, verbal and physical, at school and toward her parents.

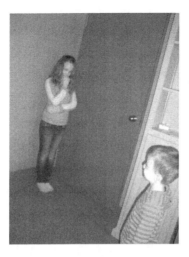

Figure 9.4 Siblings Negotiate Boundaries

Interestingly, she was not physically aggressive to her other mother (she had lesbian parents). The birth mother often attended sessions with her daughter.

We conducted a boundary experiment using yarn. After engaging mother and daughter in a body scan, I invited them to create their personal boundaries. We were in a large room so they had a lot of space. I watched as the adolescent moved to the far end of the room, where she created a boundary around herself with the yarn. Her mother then took her yarn and made an enormous circle that encompassed her daughter. As mother created her boundary, her daughter's eyes widened and her body stiffened. She later reported that she held her breath for a moment as well. Once they were finished with creating their boundaries, we engaged in discussion about their experience of the boundaries as laid out. The mother was surprised to learn that her daughter did not like being in her mother's space. They were able to identify and share somatic indicators of their discomfort and went on to navigate healthier mother–adolescent boundaries.

- Experimenting with personal space with hula hoops and the Too Close, Too Far, Just Right game (listed in Appendix B). Games are more useful for engaging younger children in exploration and experimentation with boundaries and personal space.
- Nonverbal boundaries – saying "no" with the body. See Figure 9.5. Based on Ogden & Fisher (2015), I created an activity with laminated cards for youth to practice nonverbal boundary-setting. Through role-play (in mindfulness so that they can report their current experience through the building blocks), youth practice setting boundaries with gesture with hands or arms, taking on an assertive posture, and using the eyes and facial expressions.

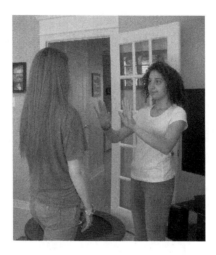

Figure 9.5 Adolescents Practice Setting Boundaries by Saying No with Their Bodies

Case Illustration

Kevin

Kevin was a 10-year-old boy who had witnessed interpersonal violence between his parents. Additionally, his mom suffered with clinical depression and often appeared frightened. Neither caregiver was attuned to this boy. Kevin's father was no longer in the family home and Kevin had very little contact with him. Kevin learned early in life that he could not depend on his mother to meet his needs, yet he depended on her for his very survival. Core beliefs that he developed about himself and others were reflected in his movements and posture. He made no effort to reach out to or connect with others, and there was no visible interest in seeking proximity with his caregiver.

In earlier sessions, Kevin typically began with his back to me as he engaged in aggressive (reenactment) play with figures in a dollhouse. Initially I sat away from him, giving him space. Because of the strategies he had developed to maintain relationship (e.g. not appear vulnerable or needy, monitor the mood of others to determine how he should react, and an awareness that he has to take care of others in order to survive and stay connected to attachment figures), he was given lots of freedom and choice about level of interaction in sessions. Over time, he invited me to play with him. Initially, he reveled in attacking my figures in the dollhouse. Using prosody and nonverbal communication, I provided interactive regulation. Over time, he stopped attacking my figures and his body appeared to soften. We moved to more interactive, prosocial games such as rolling a soft ball across the floor. Kevin's first impulse was to throw the ball hard in the therapist's direction; he did that a few times with boisterous laughter. His inability to set boundaries and determine how and when he sought proximity was evident in his shift from disengagement to aggressive behavior. He was eventually able to slow himself down as we developed a rhythm in playful activity. Being in an attuned relationship an unfamiliar person may have evoked sympathetic arousal without the social engagement system online to temper his fight response. Ultimately, Kevin exhibited comfort in setting his boundaries and personal space, his social engagement behaviors increased (e.g. eye contact, smiling/greater range of affect), and his posture became more aligned.

10 Movement and Posture

The nervous system is occupied mainly with movement.
(Moshe Feldenkrais, 1990)

Through movement the fetus, infant, child, and adult continually learn about themselves, others, and the world in an ongoing interactive dance.
(Pat Ogden, 2017)

Movement occurs on many levels, both within and outside our conscious awareness. Our movements, gestures, and posture are developed and reinforced through our earlier experiences, and they reflect our beliefs about ourselves, others, and the world. Sensorimotor Psychotherapy™ (SP) works directly with the patterns of movement, posture, and gestures to uncover the entrenched beliefs (Ogden & Fisher, 2015). The SP clinician helps the client acknowledge and honor the adaptive function these patterns have played for the child's survival, while assisting her to explore and change the patterns to reflect her current, presumably safe, life situation. As noted in Chapter 4, it is advisable that the youth be in a safe home environment before commencing this work. The traumatized child's sense of safety is often reflected in their movements and posture. For example, the child may have developed a posture that helped him feel safe in a home with domestic violence, and his body continues to hold this form despite living in a safe home with no violence around him. Aposhyan (2004) asserts that we can form initial hypotheses about the organization of the body by observing movement, breath, voice tone, and posture. Since there are so many facets to posture and movement, which serve as entry points for clinical work, they are expounded separately. We are often working concurrently with more than one facet. Also, we shall learn more about working with movement and posture through case illustrations. Finally, specific interventions and strategies to engage youth in working with posture and movement are offered.

Alignment/Lengthening the Spine

Alignment is one of the first areas I explore with traumatized youth. Alignment can, literally, bring the nervous system back into alignment or homeostasis. As

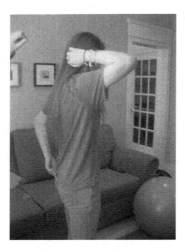

Figure 10.1 Adolescent Creates Concrete Reminder of Alignment/Lengthening the Spine to Include in Her Toolkit

the clinician remains playful and curious, and models the movements with the youth, we try out different alignments of the spine and notice how they impact various aspects such as our breathing, areas of tension, and our view of self and others. Changing alignment by lengthening the spine allows us to breathe into places we might not normally breathe (Doctor, 2018).

Since this is explored early in treatment, there is no touch involved. Instead, I have created an activity whereby I ask the youth to select from an assortment of colored bead strings. A note of caution: we need to be sure the youth is comfortable with us standing behind them prior to engaging in the activity. Once they select their color, we measure the length to match their spine (see Figure 10.1). This is done by holding one end up to the child's neck/head, then she takes it from me and positions it at the top of her spine/base of her skull. Next, I offer the other end near the tailbone a few inches from her body, and invite her to take that and position it at her tailbone. The string of beads is then custom cut to fit. This serves as a concrete reminder of the alignment activities engaged in earlier, and the benefits of having an aligned spine. The alignment beads are often the first item youth put into their coping skills/regulation toolkits. An illustration of working with alignment with Dee appears at the end of this chapter.

Rhythm

Rhythm is a fundamental ingredient to human survival. Rhythm is involved in the regulation of basic processes such as heart rate and sleep patterns. Infants are born with the ability to use rhythm for self-expression (Trevarthen, Delafield-Butt & Schögler, 2011). If a child experiences early neglect or trauma, these capacities may be truncated. As Perry (2006) asserts, we cannot survive "if our bodies cannot keep the most fundamental rhythm of life – the heartbeat" (p. 142). It is easy to imagine how rhythm may be impacted by complex trauma and neglect. For example, if the child is in a constant state of hypervigilance or high arousal, there will be increased heart rate. Over time, this high activation becomes the norm and this increases the potential for physical and mental health problems (see ACEs study for details). If the child lives in a chaotic household, and there is inconsistency and unpredictability, brain development may reflect that chaos, resulting in underdevelopment (or uneven development) of the lower, critical brain areas.

The good news is we have a multitude of ways to introduce rhythm into our clinical work to promote the rewiring or reorganization of the brain (thanks again to neuroplasticity!). Two methods to enhance rhythm are described separately within this chapter – dance and yoga – but there is also music, drumming, and singing, to name a few. Breathwork, increasing awareness and control of, is an important tool in the service of (and beneficiary of) incorporating rhythm. Note that breathwork, detailed in Chapter 8, is central to self-regulation. Perry and Hambrick (2006) emphasize the importance of using "patterned, repetitive somatosensory activities" (p. 42) to address concerns such as impulsivity and dysregulated affect associated with the poorly developed lower brain areas. There is research suggesting that performance of music, such as drumming and percussion rather than just listening, has a greater impact on improving the client's well-being (Yap, Ang & Kwan, 2017). Because children and youth enjoy play and novel activities, I keep a variety of rhythm-generating tools in my office. For example, clients can choose from a djembe, singing bowl, tambourine, gong, bongos, a rainstick, and maracas. Many of these instruments have multiple uses, such as inducing feelings of calm simply by listening to the sound, or enhancing a sense of competence by mastering the instrument. Additionally, I may ask them if there is music they might like to listen to as we move through the session, providing rhythm in the background that tends to put the youth at ease. It is judicious to have a variety to choose from since individual youth will have their own desired sounds and movements. We can also simply tap or stomp our feet with them. These activities also build play and curiosity, capacities often lost in adverse childhood experiences. As Geller (2009) notes: "Drumming is an ancient indigenous technology that uses the twin realities of rhythm and sound to bring about alignment of body, mind and spirit." (p. 12).

Foundational Developmental Movements

From birth through infancy, the foundational actions of yield, push, reach, grasp, and pull are developed. Although the process is not entirely linear, one builds upon the other as the child grows and interacts with their caregiver and the environment. Bainbridge-Cohen has created a program, Body–Mind Centering (BMC), which explores the foundational actions through movement. Others, such as Susan Aposhyan (Body–Mind Psychotherapy), have expanded on BMC to increase applicability to the psychotherapy realm. Deirdre Faye notes:

Yielding is about allowing in, letting others affect us; pushing we keep away, we develop protective boundaries, appropriate separation when needed; reach is about that reaching for, asking, wanting, needing; grasp is about clinging, holding on; and pull is about bringing others to us, connecting in a physical, emotional way.

(SafelyEmbodied.com, Summer Seminar 2015)

When an infant yields, she learns to relax her body on a physiological level, enabling her to take in the nourishment and love offered by her caregiver. The capacity to yield reflects activation of the parasympathetic nervous system, or our rest and digest functions. The ability to let go and trust others is important in subsequent relationships. Ogden (2017) notes that "yield is a restful, alert state that encompasses qualities of receptivity, trust, surrender, and taking in of nourishment. It pertains to being rather than doing." (p. 117). Being, for someone who has had to remain alert for possible danger or engage in activities to elicit the attention or care of an attachment figure, is unfathomable. If an infant has not been able to yield in safety, she may grow up lacking the capacity for vulnerability that is central to intimate, trusting relationships.

Push allows the infant to create space or set boundaries between herself and another person. According to Ogden (2017), "the pushing action asserts our will, and is often associated with the word 'no' that facilitates not only protection, but also differentiation, self-identity and self-support." (p. 119). If the baby is feeling too much stimulation or a sense of intrusiveness by the caregiver, he can push away with his arms or body. If the caregiver responds in an accepting way, the baby learns that he can set boundaries and remain connected to loved ones. If, however, the attempt to create a boundary is met with punishment or the refusal to allow space, the baby may internalize a belief that he must set aside his own needs in order to stay connected to the attachment figure. Differentiation is a developmental task that may be truncated due to early quashing of the child's efforts to assert himself with pushing actions.

Reach is about getting needs met. If the baby reaches out for something, or for connection, and this is responded to in a positive manner, she learns that it is okay to have needs and that it is okay to reach out in order to have those needs met. Grasping enables the infant to hang onto or cling to the caregiver. This may be necessary in times of distress when the infant is seeking soothing through the proximity to her caregiver (co-regulation). If the caregiver rejects or dismisses the infant's attempt to hang on for a period of time, she may learn that connections are short-lived. Further, she may either abandon this action, or she may develop a tendency to continually seek attachment figures that accept her need to stay close.

Pull involves reaching out to pull someone or something desirable closer to you. The baby may want someone close to feel safer, or they may reach and pull the squeaky toy closer to provide needed stimulation. The latter example with the toy is a baby self-regulating, but she would have learned and practiced this capacity through her initial relationship with the caregiver. We can surmise how these forms of connecting to others, and receiving an affirming response, can enhance a child's ability to connect to others; conversely, absent, negative, or inconsistent responses may increase a child's vulnerability to various forms of abuse.

The developmental movements are experienced and strengthened through relationship with a trusted other. Youth who have not had the opportunity to learn, practice, and embody these movements may face challenges in their capacity to regulate through relationship with others. For example, an infant's body naturally yields, as it has not yet learned to be armored or defend itself against threat. Defensive responses develop over time via dyadic relationships with caregivers. A healthy individual possesses the abilities to both co- and auto-regulate. So how do we work somatically with youth lacking these capacities and, further, how do we help caregivers develop the capacity to coregulate their children?

The first step is to observe the youth's movements and the patterned behaviors, posture, and gestures as they arise in sessions. We also observe the caregiver's tendencies and the interplay between them. Do the child's arms hang limply at his sides? Do his neck and head move back slightly when his father sits down next to him? Does he curl inward, pressing his body into the corner of the couch whenever his mother enters the room? Does he cross his arms over his chest when his foster mother attempts to hug him? Does he appear to be reaching forward with his body and eyes toward his mother sitting across the room? It helps us to be curious and make mental notes of these tendencies as they arise early in treatment so that we may share our observations at a later time when there is a trusting relationship between clients and therapist. We are not interpreting what we see but we are cataloging observations in order to explore and work with them somatically later.

Orienting

A child who has repeatedly faced threat or witnesses frightening events can develop a propensity to attend to reminders of these experiences. For example, keeping your eyes on (or orienting to) the door becomes a way to cope with expectations of danger. Orienting occurs on an unconscious level. As the danger abates, however, and the child continues to keep her eyes focused on the door, there can be challenges in situations that require her attention, such as learning in school or fully engaging in social interaction. As Ogden and Fisher (2015) explicate: "Clients who fail to orient toward real dangers in the environment or who hyperorient to reminders of past trauma might discover a correlation between their orienting habits and symptoms such as fight-flight responses, depression, cutting, or other types of self-harm." (p. 112). Thus, as she orients toward anticipated danger based on past experiences, she may actually miss cues of real threat.

Tracking our client's orienting habits is the first step, and then we can experiment with reorienting. Does he appear more attentive with certain proximity or prosody? Does his body tense and his gaze lock on you when talking about a particular topic? Is her head tilted in a particular direction, or does her gaze return to certain directions or objects in the room? These are things to explore and contact (reflect on and bring to client awareness) in treatment. Once the client is aware, we can explore the experience (sensation, thoughts, feelings, etc.) of orienting to and away from the object or direction.

Directed orienting activities are useful when a client is triggered, such as during a flashback or a state of dissociation. I use a modified version of Dolan's (1991) 54321 technique to help bring the youth back into the room, to orient to the present time and space:

> Look around the room and tell me three things you see. *(If they do not turn their heads, I suggest that they look at the other side of the room too, thus breaking a pattern to orient to or away from a particular direction.)*
>
> Ok, now tell me three things you hear. *(This can be difficult in a quiet office space so reassure them that it is okay to take their time if they are having difficulty.)*
>
> Ah, ok, now tell me three things you feel. *(If the client appears confused, and they sometimes do, give an example like, "your hand on the pillow." The client might identify emotions, so we want to ensure they connect to tactile sensations as well.)*
>
> Repeat the instructions above: two things you see, hear, feel; then one thing you see, hear, and feel. Again, if the room is devoid of sound, let them know they can repeat for sounds.

If necessary, reorienting is done in the moment to bring the client back from a dissociative state. Otherwise, I teach this technique early in treatment as part of phase one (safety and stabilization) to clients who have a tendency to dissociate or get triggered into flashbacks, and I suggest that they practice when they are not feeling distressed so that it comes easily to them when they need it. The analogies of practicing before you are able to tie shoelaces or ride a bike without thinking about what you are doing are helpful to get youth on board with the practice piece. I might also suggest that they put a soothing image or object near the bed so they can orient to it at bedtime or upon wakening from a nightmare (also, see Rothschild's protocols in Chapter 8).

The Feldenkrais Method (FM)

Feldenkrais wrote "breathing is movement" (1990, p. 37). Breathing, a brain stem regulated function, occurs below our level of consciousness so we are often not aware if we have stopped breathing. For example, how many times have we been driving in heavy traffic or engrossed in a book passage and then realized that we were barely breathing? We are more inclined to notice our fast breathing, such as when in a state of fight or flight, than our slowed or stuck breath. There are many ways to explore and work with breath;

however, I am going to focus here on the Feldenkrais Method (FM). I was really drawn to the similarities between FM, SP, and Hakomi: gentle, collaborative, mind–body–spirit holism, and holistic. With FM, we can have a practitioner gently manually manipulate us, and we can learn and practice the movements on our own. I was fortunate to connect with a skilled FM practitioner and she granted me an interview about the use of FM with trauma survivors. Following is an edited portion of a transcript from an interview I had with Fariya Doctor, a Feldenkrais practitioner in the Niagara Region. Doctor identified four ways we can work with traumatized clients to alter habitual patterned responses.

> With someone in a freeze place, start with them sensing their breath, where they're breathing and not breathing. Sometimes the ribs get really still and the lungs don't have room for movement. Help them with visuals, imagery of something pleasing as a way in. They can manipulate themselves, I don't do it, they do it at the start.
>
> Try stimulating the idea of a long exhale because often they're not getting the air out either. So there are different ways go get that vagal tone. Ujjayi breathing, for example. It's a noisy exhale through the throat, narrowing to get a long, slow breath.
>
> To get out of a freeze response, we can also use the eyes in a non-habitual way. With freeze, the eyes are often fixed. Start with getting them to do slow blinking. This quiets the nervous system. You feel the eyelids cover and open over the eye; often blinking can be staccato and there's a lot of tension around the eyes. They might notice that one eye closes faster. Ask them to notice what happens to the breath, do the eyeballs move up or down as they slowly blink?
>
> Have the eyes track with the head. So if there's trauma, someone might not like looking a certain way; we don't have them turn the head but you might ask them to turn the eyes only, or their eyes and head in opposite directions. Because it's non-habitual, you pay a lot of attention to that organization because it may not be easy. Anything you do that's non-habitual takes them out of the familiar state.
>
> Backwards walking slowly, feeling each foot, being really clear about landing on each foot, feeling balanced on each foot. And, suddenly having to pay attention to what's behind you, sensing that the wall is coming up. These non-habitual activities help with freeze.
>
> Lying on their back with feet in standing position [see Figure 10.2], have them stomp with each foot one at a time and make a sound. Have them pick up one foot maybe an inch, and drop it like dead weight. They are creating sound, force, and oscillation. Then maybe both feet at once two inches up and drop them, if they are able. This creates bounce in the system, it's a bit playful and gets them to loosen up in the body. It's about any way you can get in to feel the skeleton, and feel the spine, and stimulate movement, to help people get back into their body. And, feel the relationship not just with the skin but also with the web and the connections

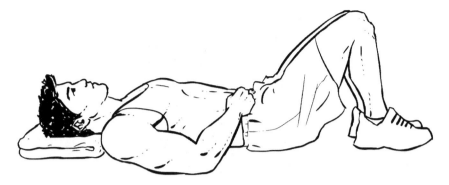

Figure 10.2 Lying on Back with Feet in Standing Position
Source: William Artamon, WorkoutLabs. Image used with permission.

within the body. It allows them to feel the connections between bones, it's novel, and often people giggle.

One of the principles of Feldenkrais is to help people feel safe and comfortable. When you start working with someone, you're checking in with them to ensure they feel comfortable (and pain-free). The idea is when you feel safe, you're more available to learn, and when you're more available to learn, changes happen more readily. The nervous system can attend to what the therapist is offering: when you quiet the body down, there's more receptivity for learning. The contact is gentle, a listening touch, and the parasympathetic nervous system is more activated. Clients notice their stomach is gurgling as the digestive system kicks in. With Feldenkrais, nothing is imposed. New movements are offered in a way that the person finds interesting and non-threatening. We are sensitive that there may be underlying trauma causing the pain.

Since my first Feldenkrais experience, I wondered how FM could be incorporated into my work with traumatized youth. As Doctor noted above, movement or activity, such as slowly blinking the eyes or walking backwards, takes the client out of the patterned response or state. Youth have been receptive to the slowly walking backwards exercise, done initially in the office and then sometimes assigned as practice between sessions, and they report increased fluidity in their bodies and fuller breaths. A breath activity that I like to introduce to young clients involves standing, lengthening and softly stretching the body, then breathing into areas that the client might not have breathed before (see Figure 10.3). Youth are fascinated when their chests are expanded and they notice the breath flowing into the upper chest corners. For extra benefit, and if the client can do so without discomfort, ask them to look over their opposite shoulder as they breathe into it. Adding a color to the breath helps facilitate the flow of breathing and makes it more interesting, especially for visual learners. There is more on FM in Doidge's latest book, *The Brain's Way of Healing:*

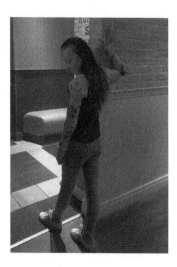

Figure 10.3 Adolescent Girl Uses an Expansive Feldenkrais Posture to Enhance Breathing Capacity

Remarkable Discoveries and Recoveries from the Frontiers of Neuroplasticity (2015).

Note: for breathwork with youth, we can use cards from the Yoga Pretzels deck (see details in Appendix B). I also like to use a balloon to demonstrate the difference between breathing quickly and slowly. Fast breathing is like letting go of the air-filled balloon and watching it shoot out of control around the room. When we hold the end of the balloon and release air slowly, it is smooth and controlled. I equate this to us maintaining a semblance of control over ourselves (thoughts, feelings, behaviors) when we are mindful of our breath.

Rosenberg's (2017) *Accessing the Healing Power of the Vagus Nerve* does not mention FM but contains similar movements and activities with a focus on the vagus nerve. One of Rosenberg's self-help exercises that youth have been willing to learn in session and then practice between sessions is the "half-salamander" exercise. Perhaps youth like the simplicity of the exercise, or maybe they like the name, as youth are more receptive to activities with playful or fun names. The salamander exercise "contributes to the freedom of movement of your ribs and promotes optimal breathing." (p. 200). These are Rosenberg's (2017, pp. 200–201) instructions for the half-salamander exercise:

> Client may be seated or standing in a comfortable position for the first part of the Salamander Exercise. *(Note: I usually invite youth to do this exercise in a seated position because they find it more comfortable than standing.)*

1. Let your eyes look to the right without turning your head.
2. Continue to face forward, begin tilting your head to the right so that your right ear moves closer to your right shoulder. Make this movement without lifting your right shoulder toward your ear. Hold this position for about 30 seconds.
3. Return your head to neutral position, then allow your eyes to look straight ahead again.
4. Repeat steps 1–3 with the other side (e.g. eyes to the left, side-bend head, hold position about 30 seconds, then return head to upright position and eyes facing forward).

Qigong

Qigong was developed in China over 4,000 years ago. "Qi" means vital energy and "gong" can be interpreted as mastery or cultivation. The practice involves slow, repetitive movements intended to enhance health and well-being. There is some research to support the use of qigong in improving health conditions such as hypertension and arthritis (Lee et al., 2007; Marks, 2017). While many styles of qigong exist, there is usually a focus on breath, and increasing flow of energy along meridians (internal pathways associated with specific organs of the body, like the kidney and lungs). Personally, I began qigong classes a few years ago, and I have continued my own personal practice. As always, I wondered how to integrate qigong into my clinical work with traumatized youth given that I am not trained and thus I am not authorized to instruct clients in the use of qigong.

A couple of years ago I stumbled across a series of videos on YouTube. Lee Holden offers 10 and 20-minute guided practices in a way that is clear and enjoyable. I appreciate his soothing prosody and modifications for varying levels of mobility, and I share these videos with clients of all ages. I found that younger children and teens enjoy the shorter morning clips, while young adults seem to gravitate toward the short evening clips. The morning practices are about energizing the body and gaining mental clarity, and the evening practices focus on letting go of the day's stress and relaxing the mind and body. Children especially like the names of some of the fun, simple moves, such as "embrace the tiger/return to the mountain" and "water waves." See the images in Figures 10.4 and 10.5 of a young boy moving through a centering qigong movement sequence. Of course, be sure to check in with your client before and throughout about any pain during the movements, and go through the movements with your client. If they like a particular movement, we could integrate it into our sessions, for example before we begin or as we close.

1. Begin with both hands sitting in front of the stomach area, palms upward.
2. As you inhale, bring your right arm out and up as though scooping up good energy, until your hand is up over your head. Your hand should be straight with your fingertips pointing upward (as in Figure 10.5 but up over your head).

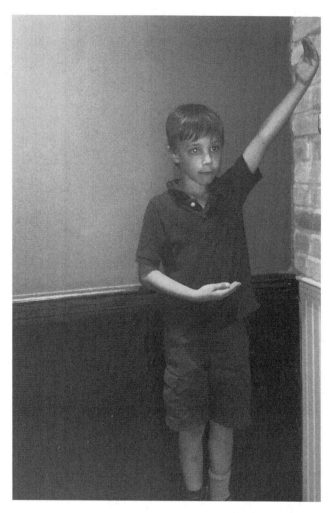

Figure 10.4 A Young Boy Practices Qigong Centering Movements

3. Bring your hand down in front of your body as you exhale fully, your right hand placed slightly above the left.
4. Repeat steps 1–3 with the left arm. Do this movement exercise 3–5 times for each arm.

Lee Holden on centering:

> In terms of Qi Gong, centering means having energy in the center of the body, also known as Dan Tien. Energy is stored in the center of the body and can be viewed as a place of inner strength. Following is one of Lee Holden's centring qi gong exercises that focuses on breathing:

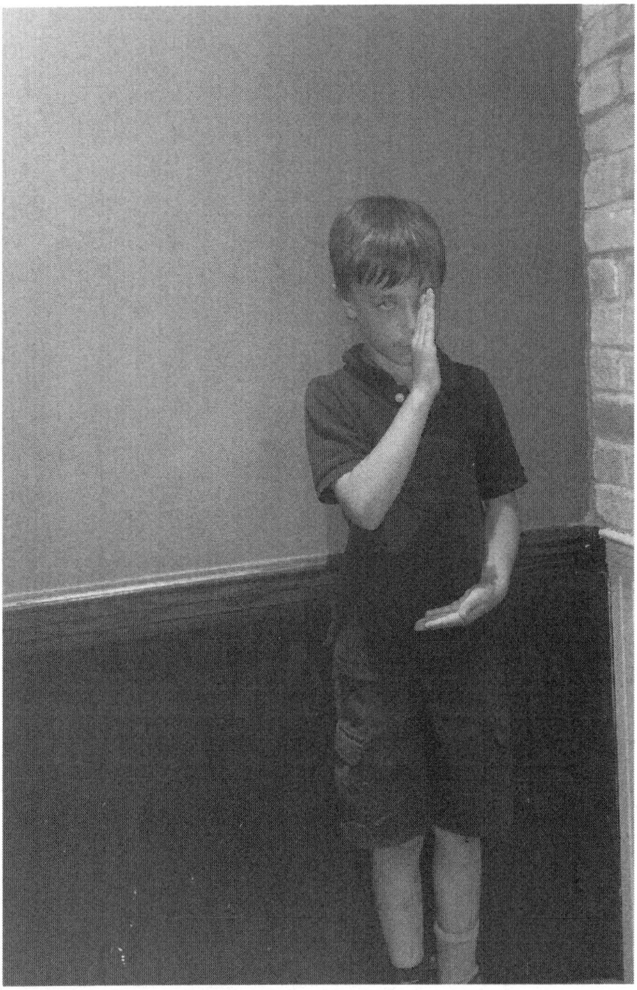

Figure 10.5 A Young Boy Practices Qigong Centering Movements

Exercise: Deep Abdominal Breathing (Dan Tien Breathing)

1. Sit in a chair with the spine straight and bring both hands over the lower abdomen.
2. Breathe in and out through the nose. Breathing through the nose helps to cultivate more "qi" out of the air.
3. Then, inhale down into the lower abdomen so that the belly expands. This allows the diaphragm to relax and air to move into the deeper areas of the lungs.

4. Exhale, all the way out to clear the lungs. During "normal" breathing, we usually only exhale 40% of the air out, which leaves little room to take in a deep breath. So, at the bottom of your exhale, see if you can exhale a little more.
5. Again, exhale and squeeze the air out from the lower abdomen.
6. Then, take in a full deep breath down into the lower abdomen.
7. During this breathing exercise, keep the chest relaxed.
8. Visualize a golden ball of energy, like a small sun, growing in your lower Dan Tien. With each breath see this light growing brighter and brighter.
9. Practice for at least 3–5 minutes (10 minutes is ideal). Throughout the day, take one or two Dan Tien breaths to recharge your internal energy.
10. Enjoy.

Source: Used with permission: www.leeholden.com/ announcements/connecting-to-the-center. Lee Holden. More information at www.holdenqigong.com

There is an abundance of research and books written on the benefits of trauma-sensitive yoga (see, for example, Emerson, 2015; Fay, 2017; van der Kolk et al., 2014). I have only recently begun venturing in the world of yoga for myself, and I have experienced its benefits in terms of movement and posture. Yoga works with the breath, slow extended movements, and moves us into positions we would not normally move thereby. There is an inherent rhythm through the repetitive movements and awareness of breath that calms the nervous system. For most of us, yoga introduces movements that are not habituated and thus can bring about positive change. Though the practice of yoga is new to me, I have been using Yoga Pretzels (listed with the resources in Appendix B) with young traumatized clients for many years. In the deck is a card that invites youth to create five poses that represent natural phenomena. For example, they might say wind, rain, tree, sunshine, and tornado. After they create the pose, they demonstrate and hold it for five seconds. As part of the playful process, I ask that they not include any positions on the floor because it might be difficult for me to get back up – youth frequently enjoy doing exactly that! I often have to remind them to breathe as they sustain the pose. This is a playful, creative way to engage youth in movement and self-expression, and provides an opportunity for enhancing mastery and competence. The latter point shines through when the youth invite their caregiver in to demonstrate the poses they created. Often the youth and caregiver agree to practice at home together at the start or end of their days. Many caregivers have reported that they have found this practice helpful in terms of their own self-regulation. General yoga poses, such as the warrior pose, the cat pose, or other animal poses, are more appealing to young children. Adolescents report that the warrior pose is empowering. There are abundant resources for integrating yoga, in book, card game, and video formats, available for clinicians. See Appendix B for selected yoga pose resources.

Let's Dance!

There is plenty of research on the use of therapeutic dance with trauma survivors. A recently published review article suggests a dance/movement therapy model, focusing on interoception, to treat trauma survivors (Dieterich-Hartwell, 2017). Interoception is the awareness of what is happening in the body, such as noticing that you are hungry. Clinicians who use dance or movement in their work are drawn to somatic psychotherapeutic methods because they see the benefits in their clients. As one clinician stated, "I have seen that both movement and dance provide the opportunity to discover or recover spontaneous expressions or gesture, to experience the witnessing of the self and other, to mindfully notice and feel a deepening or more integrated experience of sensation and emotion" (Miriam Schacter, personal communication). Dancing is also often a social activity and thus provides opportunity for interactive regulation. I remember working with one girl many years ago that used visual arts and dance to create and share her TF-CBT trauma narrative. The dance piece was at the end of the narrative and, for her, it symbolized empowerment and movement beyond her trauma. Her father, a single dad who fought for years to get custody of his daughter from her abusive mother, was moved to tears as he watched her share her story.

Case Illustrations

Dee

During our first meeting, I noticed that Dee's posture was slumped and her chest collapsed as she sat on the couch across from me. Her head hung slightly forward. Eye contact was good from the start. Over the course of the assessment, I learned that Dee liked art and music and these were both important to her, especially music. She had her headphones on when she arrived in and left the office every session. We began bringing her music into the office, and Dee shared her favorite songs and bands. When listening to music and creating art, there was a soft flow to her movement not otherwise observed, and Dee's posture was less slumped. I contacted this: "Dee, I've noticed that you sit more upright and there's a little rocking motion when you listen to your music. Did you ever notice that?" Dee responded that she had not and agreed to experiment with posture/alignment.

K: So let's start by just noticing your breath, any areas of tension, sensations, or whatever else you notice when you sit on the couch. Just like a body scan from head to toe.
D: Yeah, I don't really notice anything.
K: What about your breath? Do you notice your breath?
D: Uh, yah, I guess so. (*shrugs shoulders and raises eyebrows quizzically*)

K: I wonder if you could describe your breath for me, like the quality of your breathing. Is it fast, slow, is it short or full?

D: Hmmmm, short, slow.

K: I'm curious about what might change if we sort of align our spines, you know, lengthen it like we have an invisible string at the top of our heads pulling us upward a little. *(I point to the top of my head and demonstrate by lifting my chin slightly. Dee watches then follows my movement.)* As we do this, let's try to relax our shoulders, too, down and back. *(Again, I model this in a slightly exaggerated manner with dropping the shoulders on the exhalation, noting that the exhale is when the relaxation occurs.)* So, what do you notice? Anything change with your breathing? Maybe, maybe not.

D: I think it's a little fuller, like not just in this area of my chest. *(She makes a circular motion in the center of her chest.)*

K: Well, isn't that interesting. I wonder if we could hang out like this for a while, just noticing our breathing as we keep sitting like this.

D: Ok.

I turned the music back on and, after a few minutes, Dee noted that her back and shoulders were hurting. It makes sense that she might experience discomfort since her muscles, bones, and organs were unaccustomed to this posture. She resumed her usual posture for the remainder of the session. We repeated this experiment in subsequent sessions, and added walking mindfully to embody the posture. Additionally, we explored the thoughts, feelings, and sensations that went along with each of the postures (slumped, lengthened spine). Note: Dee also suffered from digestive problems, not uncommon with constricted breathing. She did not eat regular, healthy meals and this certainly contributed to her digestive issues, but there was some improvement over time after she practiced the mindful walking and attended to her breathing patterns.

Kevin

Kevin usually entered the room with a sort of shuffling movement of his feet. He had a slim build and his shoulders were drawn upward as though he were in a state of preparation or expectation. While he moved forward, there was a slight leaning back from his waist and his head was somewhat tilted to one side. His eyes were often round and wide but there was limited eye contact. When I observed Kevin's breath, it appeared to be short and shallow in his upper chest.

Kevin responded well to being given choices of activity for the session, rather than having something imposed on him. Aware that he was vigilant, I was mindful of my prosody, proximity, and movements around him. I was especially mindful of where I was in relation to his gaze since his head was slightly tilted to one side. I later learned that he was frequently in his room with his sister when the abuse between his parents occurred, with his head oriented to the door to his left. We experimented (played) with movement and proximity: I rolled my chair away from him and asked him to check in with how this affected him (e.g. his breathing, the neck, and overall tension). Offered a choice of musical instruments, Kevin chose a set of bongos. After he tapped lightly on them for a while, I invited him to makes sounds that reflected his feelings, any feelings he might have at the moment. Kevin drummed out three feelings: angry, sad, and bored. I watched him and observed his breath with each feeling, then checked in with him about his breath. He noticed that his breath changed following the drumming pattern. I then asked if we could play together and he agreed. First I followed his lead, then we took turns. Kevin was able to maintain a relational connection through the drumming, and at times a small smile curled at the corner of his mouth. Eventually we were drumming together in a slower rhythm: I observed that as Kevin's shoulder tension settled, color appeared in his face and there was more fluidity to his movement. We discussed the experience afterward and explored ways Kevin could carry this practice into his home life.

The experiments were titrated and woven into other activities as Kevin was sensitive to perceived threat and oriented toward signs of potential threat. As an animal rescuer, I have seen this fear/freeze response in animals many times. Play was completely off the table initially with Kevin, but as he felt safer and engaged in rhythmic, empowering activities, his body relaxed, his gait grew lighter, his posture straightened, and his body appeared less disjointed. Additionally, the tilt in Kevin's neck was diminished as his body experienced a safe, attuned presence.

Part IV

Special Populations

11 LGBTQ+ Youth

The challenge of being lesbian, gay, bisexual or transgendered is difficult enough to manage for someone who has not been traumatized in childhood. That challenge is exponentially increased when the individual is also struggling with a history of sexual abuse.

(Margo Rivera, 2002)

While not wishing to further "other" LGBTQ+ youth, this section is separate to highlight the additional challenges faced by LGBTQ+ youth with histories of childhood trauma and neglect. In this chapter, LGBTQ+ stands for lesbian, gay, bisexual, transgender, queer, plus. Note that the plus includes other sexual minorities such as intersex, two-spirited, asexual, pansexual, and gender-nonconforming and nonbinary individuals. A chart containing LGBTQ+ terms is included at the end of this chapter for reference purposes. The correlation between increased mental health issues, such as depression, anxiety, self-injury, and suicidal ideation, and LGBTQ+ is well documented (see, for example, Hottes et al., 2016). Clinicians with experience working with traumatized LGBTQ+ youth are aware of the associated health issues, and research has begun to examine the relationship between adverse childhood experiences and higher incidence of mental and physical health issues in LGBTQ+ adults (Andersen, Zou & Blosnich, 2015; Austin, Herrick & Proescholdbell, 2015; Roberts et al., 2010). The past few years have seen a growing body of research addressing increased health issues among LGBTQ+ youth with a history of adverse childhood experiences (Becerra-Culqui et al., 2018; Mustanski, Garofalo & Emerson, 2010; National Child Traumatic Stress Network, 2014). Following is a discussion of the various risk factors that are unique to this client population, protective factors, and suggested ways we can improve our clinical work with traumatized LGBTQ+ youth.

ACEs Research

Research using the ACEs (adverse childhood experiences) scale identifies higher rates of adverse childhood experiences among LGBTQ+ adults compared to heterosexuals (Andersen & Blosnich, 2013; Zou & Andersen, 2015). Zou & Andersen (2015) found that LGBTQ+ individuals are 60% more likely to have a history of some form of childhood trauma than the heterosexual population. Also consistent with adult research, Clements-Nolle and colleagues (2018) found that LGBTQ+ youth are more likely to witness domestic violence in the home, and more likely to live with an adult experiencing substance abuse or mental health issues. ACEs include verbal or physical abuse, sexual abuse, physical or emotional neglect, household dysfunction (e.g. living with a caregiver with a mental illness), and school bullying. A large American study of over 10,000 LGBTQ-identified youth between 13 and 17 years of age, conducted by the Human Rights Campaign Foundation in 2012, indicates that sexual minority youth are twice as likely to report having been verbally harassed at school compared to their heterosexual peers.

The consequences of adverse childhood experiences include greater risk of self-injury, suicidal ideation, mood disturbance, and use of substances (alcohol, drugs, cigarettes). Given these high numbers, one might leap to the assumption that the LGBTQ+ identity stems from the early childhood trauma; however, as we know, not all traumatized children grow up to identify as LGBTQ+. As clinicians, we need to be aware of the increased prevalence of early childhood trauma among LGBTQ+ youth and explore the possibility of these experiences during the assessment process, and we must include interventions that target the potential consequences. Furthermore, there is a dose-response relationship between the number of ACEs and likelihood of long-term health issues such as heart disease, liver disease, and respiratory conditions.

Risk Factors for Trauma in LGBTQ+ Youth

Being different in the school setting is generally recognized as a risk factor for bullying. Youth may be singled out for being different due to physical or cognitive impairments, or gender nonconformity. Gender nonconformity exhibited before the age of 11 is considered a risk factor for physical, psychological, and sexual abuse both at school and in the home, resulting in elevated risk for depressive symptoms (Roberts et al., 2013; Roberts et al., 2012). Beyond overt discrimination, and verbal and physical assaults, LGBTQ+ youth are frequently victims of microaggression (Briggs et al., 2018; Nadal, 2011). Microaggressions are subtler forms of discrimination which LGBTQ+ youth may experience daily. Examples of microaggression include: being stared at when walking hand-in-hand with your partner, being told "but you don't look like a lesbian" as though it were a compliment, and the still often heard expression, "That's so gay!" While gender differences and sexual orientation are both risk factors, they are not the same thing and clinicians need to be aware of the differences.

The potential for victimization increases for those both with gender differences, such as nonbinary presentation and having an orientation other than heterosexual. National Child Traumatic Stress Network (2014) highlights the difficulties for youth facing dual stigmas (i.e. both gender nonconforming and belonging to a sexual minority). To clarify terminology, transgender refers to those who identify as something different from the gender assigned at birth.

Research shows that children exhibit stable gender-typed behavior between 3 and 8 years of age (Becerra-Culqui et al., 2018). Sexual orientation refers to sexual attraction: gay, straight, bisexual, asexual, and pansexual. Thus, for example, one can be both a transman and a gay man. A comprehensive description of terms is beyond the scope of this book.

As Classen and colleagues (2005) note, a history of child sexual abuse is the best predictor of sexual revictimization, and polyvictimization in childhood further increases the risk. So, if more LGBTQ+ youth have experienced adverse childhood experiences, there is a greater risk for revictimization. Furthermore, the authors (Classen, Gronskaya Palesh & Aggarwal, 2005) indicate that areas impacted include affect regulation, coping skills, and the sense of shame. Indeed, most of my young LGBTQ+ clients experienced childhood abuse and revictimization in their adolescence, all of them struggled with affect regulation, many experienced symptoms of depression and/or anxiety, and all of them experienced a profound sense of shame. One study found that nondisclosure (i.e. not coming out) has negative effects on LBGTQ+ youth (Pereira & Rodriques, 2015). In addition to the shame and self-blame associated with having been sexually abused, the majority of my young LGBTQ+ clients experienced internalized homophobia, and internalization of the negative messages about sexual orientation (Irwin & Austin, 2013). Internalized homophobia is an additional stressor faced by LGBTQ+ youth, and more clinical attention must be paid to the relationship between internalized homophobia and suicidal ideation among LGBTQ+ youth (Bontempo & D'Augellie, 2002; Pereira & Rodrigues, 2015).

Additionally, increased risk for LGBTQ+ youth may be explained by the minority stress model. The minority stress model notes the link between an individual's chronic stress, poor health outcomes including suicidal behaviors, and membership of a stigmatized minority social group (Clements-Nolle et al., 2018; House & Stepleman, 2011). Finally, often unrecognized is the increased risk for LGBTQ+ youth to get urinary tract infections, especially gender nonconforming and trans youth. Fears of being verbally or physically assaulted prevent transgender youth from using the washrooms at school and public settings. To avoid use of public washrooms, they may refrain from drinking water and this may lead to dehydration or other health-related problems (US Transgender Survey of 2015, www.ustranssurvey.org/reports). Rates of urinary tract infections (UTIs) are high among transgender people. I have seen this avoidance and subsequent urgency to urinate when clients arrive at my office, where there is a private washroom, after having held it in for extended periods.

When I reflect on the presenting concerns of LGBTQ+ youths' caregivers, suicidal ideation and suicide attempts were common. It is worth noting here that the youth and caregivers who have called for services in my practice are caregivers that were more attuned, accepting, and nurturing than the caregivers of LGBTQ+ youth who may be homeless or, sadly, successful in their suicide attempt. While working in children's mental health agency settings, the LGBTQ+ youth with high-risk activities were typically mandated by child protection services and caregiver attunement and acceptance was not as high; however, it became a focus of treatment. It comes as no surprise, then, that LGBTQ+ individuals have a higher lifetime prevalence of self-injury and suicide attempts than do nonsexual minorities (Hottes et al., 2016; House & Stepleman, 2011; Taliaferro & Muehlenkamp, 2016), given the increased presence of the aforementioned factors (e.g. higher rates of adverse childhood experiences including victimization in home and school settings, internalized homophobia). A large-scale study by the YRBS in 2015 found that, with the inclusion of LGBTQ as an identifier, the sexual minority group was three times more likely than heterosexual youth to have experienced suicidal ideation, and nearly four times more likely to attempt suicide. Clements-Nolle and colleagues (2018) found that LGBTQ+ youth with higher ACEs had disproportionately high levels of suicidal ideation and attempts. There is also an increased risk of PTSD for LGBTQ+ individuals compared to heterosexuals (Roberts et al., 2010).

High-Risk Behaviors

Another sad reality for many LGBTQ+ youth is caregiver rejection. A very recent study by Tyler & Schmitz (2018) found that sexual minority youth are overrepresented among homeless youth and are more likely to trade sex for necessities such as food and shelter. Internalized and institutionalized homophobia make it difficult for these youth to consider shelter. Moreover, given the higher rates of childhood abuse, the likelihood of revictimization, combined with self-blame and shame experienced by sexually abused youth, these youth are more likely to resort to trading sex for survival (food, shelter, drugs/alcohol). Drugs and alcohol are frequently used by trauma survivors to self-medicate or self-soothe. In my practice, more than half of the LGBTQ+ youth assessed, mainly those between 14 and 20, reported use of alcohol and/or drugs as a coping mechanism. One study by Newcomb, Heinz and Mustanski (2012) found no differences in the pathways to alcohol use in LGBTQ+ youth compared to the general population, suggesting that similar interventions may be useful.

I am reminded of a few young gay men that I worked with who were referred by victim service agencies following sexual assaults: these young men had complex trauma histories, caregivers who rejected them, or caregivers with mental health issues or inappropriate boundaries (e.g. parentification, intrusiveness). These young men used substances regularly to cope with overwhelming emotion and viewed the trade of sex for drugs as insignificant. As we reached the sexual history section of the Time Line activity, one young man talked about his numerous sexual encounters in exchange for drugs, and he shrugged as he said, "Why not, what else was I good for?" Given the referrals were from victim service agencies, the funding was limited and we were only able to focus on phase one trauma treatment. I am also remembering one young transwoman I worked with. She had been rejected by her caregivers but was resilient, did not use substances, and she sought resources to secure housing and psychotherapy. Unfortunately, this young woman also possessed a poor self-concept, experienced severe symptoms of anxiety and depression, dysregulated affect, and she began to engage in nondiscriminatory sexual encounters as this represented affection and love for her. She was another LGBTQ+ youth referred by a local victim services agency. When the funding expired, I continued to offer sessions because her functioning had deteriorated, but she eventually stopped attending sessions and I was unable to reach her for follow-up.

Eating Disorders, Body Image Issues

LGBTQ+ youth may experience eating disorders or body image issues. In my experience, adolescent gay males, transgender girls (15–18), and young adult lesbian or bisexual women (18–25) are more likely to struggle with eating disorders and body image issues than heterosexual youth. More frequently I have observed disordered eating in the form of anorexia or restricted eating and a binge/purge cycle with young gay males than other youth. A study by Columbia University (2007) found higher rates of eating disorders among gay and bisexual men than heterosexual men. Research suggests a relationship between gender identity, sexual orientation, and eating disordered behavior (Diemer et al., 2015). The authors recommend additional research in this area as appropriate interventions are lacking. While there is overlap, there are differences between body dysmorphia and eating disorders. According to the DSM-5 (2013), body dysmorphia disorder, or BDD, involves distress related to perceived physical imperfections of a feature, such as a scar, or a body part. Eating disorders, on the other hand, involve preoccupation with the entire body (weight and shape); shame often accompanies eating disorders (Bryn Austin et al., 2009). Either may contribute to symptoms of depression among LGBTQ+ youth. The youth I have seen who are experiencing eating disordered behaviors or body image issues also present with substance use, feelings of extreme guilt and shame, dysregulated affect, and symptoms of depression and/or anxiety.

Protective Factors

Caregiver connectedness and safe school environments are seen as protective factors against self-injurious behavior and suicidality among LGBTQ+ youth (Taliaferro & Muehlenkamp, 2016). Ryan and colleagues (2010) also highlight the importance of family acceptance as a buffer against substance abuse, high-risk sexual behaviors, depression, and suicidal ideation. Additionally, LGBTQ+ youth will benefit from connection to other supportive adults and peers, community, and positive role models or mentors (National Child Traumatic Stress Network, 2014; Taliaferro & Muehlenkamp, 2016). We can facilitate referrals to youth groups or activities, and we can also provide historical information about famous LGBTQ+ individuals who overcame the odds. There is not enough awareness about positive role models and this contributes to internalized homophobia, shame, increased symptoms of depression and anxiety, and other risk factors noted above.

The therapeutic alliance has long been recognized as a critical factor in treatment effectiveness (Keating & Muller, 2018; Shirk, Karver & Brown, 2011). Keating & Muller (2018) identify therapist behaviors that enhance the effectiveness of treatment of LGBTQ+ youth with histories of trauma, including making therapy more affirming by using inclusive language, asking about pronoun preference, and having relevant symbols (e.g. pride flags, LGBTQ+ event flyers) on display in the office. Spengler et al. (2016) identified the impact of microaggressions against LGBTQ+ clients in clinical practice, and the authors recommend ongoing self-study to notice and correct therapists' biases. Choi et al. (2015) recommend that therapists be open about their non-hetero identity as this may improve the likelihood of LGBTQ+ youth seeking services. Indeed, caregivers and youth have shared that they were drawn to my services based on my website's references and openness about my sexual orientation. Positive therapy experiences have generated word-of-mouth referrals and I am honored to have the opportunity to work with these youth. With caregivers, there is often a role for psychoeducation as they express concerns about their child being victimized because they are LGBTQ+, they worry that they have done something wrong in their parenting that contributed to their youth's orientation or gender identity, and they seek direction about how to support their child. LGBTQ+ youth frequently report the positive experience of being able to talk openly with someone who accepts, supports, and "gets them."

Treatment Considerations

Given the high potential for LGBTQ+ youth to have one or more adverse childhood experiences, it makes sense for clinicians to screen for ACEs at the beginning of treatment. Screening can direct treatment interventions and reduce the likelihood of the youth further engaging in self-injurious or risky behaviors. Assessment is complicated for transgender youth because the tests are normed for males and females, and thus the results reflect either a female or a male identity. When trans youth complete psychometrics, they select their self-identified gender. Nonbinary is not an option on most assessment tools. When the results graph is produced and shared during feedback meetings, I advise them that the results may not be accurate since psychological assessment has not caught up with us. The lack of representation of nonbinary and transgender youth in assessment tools is a challenge that I am working with colleagues to rectify. Clark (2017) notes that research highlights three essential factors when it comes to transgender youth care: supporting families to support their youth, providing affirmation and support for youth, and fighting against injustices that impede the first two points. Clinicians can increase their awareness of LGBTQ+ resources in order to better direct youth to additional services (e.g. affirmative medical care, social/support groups). Clinicians need to recognize that LGBTQ+ youth are not seeking services because of their identity or gender dysphoria, but rather because of the distress they are experiencing in a stigmatizing, discriminating society. The depression and anxiety they feel are real and can be alleviated through affirmative therapy. Research has found that the mental health of transgender people improves once they receive medical treatment that is affirming of their gender, whether hormonal or surgical (Briggs, Hayes & Changaris, 2018).

Group therapy has long been recognized as a powerful intervention regardless of presenting concerns. Group treatment offers opportunities for validation and normalization of the individual's experience, enhances social engagement in a safe setting, and allows individuals to practice and master skills with peers. A couple of studies on the efficacy of Sensorimotor Psychotherapy™ (SP) informed groups with adults with Complex PTSD (Gene-Cos et al., 2016; Langmuir, Kirsh & Classen, 2012) demonstrated a reduction in PTSD symptoms and depression and improved overall health. Mark-Goldstein & Ogden (2013) found SP group work with youth enhanced self-regulation capacities and improved youths' sense of self. A small study on the utilization of Somatic Experiencing® with gender nonconforming and transgender adults had promising results (Briggs, Hayes & Changaris, 2018). In 2016, I saw the need for group work with individual LGBTQ+ clients with trauma histories, so I developed and offered a group (non-research but youth did complete pre- and post-tests). The group was co-facilitated by a trans-identified psychotherapist/artist who was in the process of SP training. Using the principles and techniques of SP, LGBTQ+ youth engaged in a 6-week group intervention. Following the group, participants reported improvements in mood, self-confidence, and ability to tolerate and manage distress. Interventions with a somatic focus, such as affect regulation and resourcing, can be effective in treatment of traumatized LGBTQ+ youth.

Case Illustrations

Dee

Dee was experimenting with her gender identity and sexual orientation when we began treatment. One of the things she wondered about was whether she was gay or bisexual because of the childhood sexual abuse. Psychoeducation addressed some of her questions. However, she also struggled with body image issues, primarily in relation to having breasts. Dee was energetic, riding around on her skateboard in a toque when she was not feeling anxiety-stricken or depressed.

Dee struggled, feeling like she was in the wrong body at times, and this was confusing. She was comfortable with sexual orientation and her caregiver and friends were accepting; however, she did not feel like she could talk about the confusion related to gender identity. The rigidity of social expectations around gender contributed to Dee's feelings of shame and self-hatred. Dee worried about not feeling or presenting as stereotypically feminine. We were able to explore the messages she received and internalized from music, social media, and television about what it meant to be female. The internalized messages contributed to

194 *Special Populations*

a negative self-concept that sometimes plummeted her into a state of despair. Learning about gender fluidity, and mindful experiments with posture and movement that felt right to her, enhanced Dee's self-concept, alleviated her reliance on stereotypical gender norms, and she reported (and appeared) increasingly comfortable in her own skin. Dee did not deviate from her toques and skateboards, but she no longer vacillated between joy and despair regarding her gender presentation.

Vincent

Vincent was 14 years old when he began treatment to address symptoms of depression and anxiety. He was referred by a local victim services program after he, along with his supportive caregivers, reported a sexual assault. Following his first assault, Vincent was revictimized sexually, and physically attacked by peers. He grew increasingly isolated, depressed, and anxious and turned to drug use to numb his emotional distress. Though Vincent was not out as a gay male at school, he experienced verbal bullying fairly regularly, and faced daily microaggressions through interaction with his teachers (e.g. homophobic comments while teaching classes) and peers and general heterosexist social messaging. Additionally, one of his older male cousins was constantly making sexual comments about women in attempts to bond or connect with Vincent in this way. These experiences left Vincent feeling deep shame and self-loathing. He was disgusted with his desires and with his body; the latter he felt had betrayed him. Vincent grew suicidal and heard voices telling him to end his life. He eventually attempted suicide and was hospitalized.

Vincent was hospitalized again shortly after his release. He was given medication that left him somnolent, labile, and noncommunicative. Vincent recalled attending individual, group, and family sessions during his hospitalizations. During the time he was hospitalized, Vincent self-identified as bisexual. He noted that his sexual orientation was omitted from individual and group discussions, like it was denied, and this intensified his sense of shame. There was a lack of communication between caregivers and hospital staff so his caregivers felt helpless to support their son. None of the treatment providers Vincent encountered to this point reported the sexual assaults. Vincent's shame and despair grew. Following his last hospitalization, Vincent was prescribed anti-depressants and anti-psychotic medication (he did not like the side effects and stopped taking the medication on his own). He was referred to a local social service agency and his social worker was the first one to validate his experience and seek victim services to address the traumatic impact.

Still, law enforcement was yet to be involved. Vincent reported feelings of hopelessness with regard to getting justice and a lack of trust in systems to meet his needs. When we began working together, Vincent presented with many distressing symptoms of Complex PTSD:

- recurrent, intrusive distressing memories of the assaults (flashbacks, frequent nightmares);
- avoidance of reminders of the assaults (places, music);
- intense physiological reactions in the form of agitation and hypervigilance;
- stomachaches and nausea alternated with feeling numb all over;
- negative mood and diminished interest in activities previously enjoyed;
- profound sense of guilt and shame;
- irritability, anger (directed at family members);
- disturbance of sleep and appetite (developed disordered eating: food restriction and occasional purging);
- negative shift in perception of himself (he hated the sight of his body, he viewed himself as disgusting because of his sexual desires);
- depersonalization (feeling detached from himself), particularly when reenacting the traumatic events.

Vincent later engaged in additional sexual activities during which he felt like he was an observer; then he would be unable to recall many of the details. His cognitive, social, emotional, and physiological functioning were impaired by the impact of his traumas. The first step with Vincent was to develop a sense of safety with an accepting, affirmative environment and therapeutic relationship. Being present and attuned to Vincent, validating his feelings and thoughts, utilizing existing resources, and providing new strategies to stay grounded and manage his physiological distress characterized the early sessions with Vincent. A harm-reduction approach was taken with his substance use. His caregivers were included in treatment when he expressed a wish to include them. Shortly after we began working together, Vincent disclosed that he had been sextorted by a peer. This disclosure became the first report to law enforcement. I observed a shift in his motivation, sense of self-efficacy, and a subsequent elevation in mood. Throughout treatment, Vincent worked through his trauma using somatic and expressive arts methods (drawing from his innate skills and interests). His trust in himself and others flourished and he began a relationship with a male peer. He developed the capacity for mindfulness and gained the ability to track himself when triggered by flashbacks so that he could return to the present moment. He began to feel safe in his body through movement, 5-sense perception and boundary exercises, and he created a toolbox of skills that he continued to use throughout treatment. Toward the end of treatment, Vincent participated in a group for LGBTQ+ youth. He was further along in treatment than the other group members and he excelled in a leadership role with his peers. He also found it incredibly affirming to be amongst LGBTQ+ peers with similar trauma experiences

Vincent was an exceptionally resilient young man who was able to heal from his traumatic experiences and went on to reach his full potential.

Although he did not have any ACEs prior to sexual victimization, he was young when the assault occurred and not sexually aware or mature, and he lived in a society that stigmatizes and discriminates against LGBTQ+ people. He was plagued with guilt and shame over what had happened to him and thus began a cascade of mental health issues and high-risk activity. Protective factors included caregiver connectedness and intelligence. Ultimately, Vincent connected with experienced clinicians who were able to assist him on his healing journey.

Vincent created masks early in treatment. He completed the outside, what he showed to the world, first. Vincent moved fairly easily and quickly through this part of the mask and appeared to enjoy his creative work. His body was relaxed and he was chatty. The colors of the outside of his mask were vibrant, with bright red lips, gold accents on the face, a reflection of happiness and joy he later said. For the inside, however, what he hid from the world, there was a different process and a very different presentation. He took time to consider how to best reflect how he felt and thought about the inside. Eventually, he glued gray-green wool all over: he felt confused, disgusted, "messy'" about his thoughts, feelings, and desires. He felt ashamed and did not want others to know about these parts of him. The inside of the mask contained no bright colors, no joy, and, most significant, he covered the mouth. During subsequent discussion, Vincent talked about feeling like he had no voice and that he dared not speak about some things. Recall that Vincent had been through several experiences (the assaults and then the service providers he encountered) where he felt unheard. The inside of his mask reflected the pain that he hid inside and the belief that his words did not matter.

An Abbreviated List of LGBTQ+ Terminology

*Asexual	People who are not sexually attracted to anyone or do not experience sexual desire.
*Bicurious	A person who is curious about having sexual contact with someone with the same gender.
*Biphobia	Fear or hatred of bisexuals – this is seen in the LGBTQ+ community as well as in general.
*Bisexual	A person physically and/or sexually, and emotionally, attracted to more than one gender.
**Cis(gender)	One who identifies with the gender they were assigned at birth.
*Gay	A man attracted to other men.
**Gender Fluid	Movement or fluidity regarding gender identity.
**Gender Identity	An individual's sense of being feminine, masculine, or another gender.
**Gender Nonconforming	When people do not adhere to social norms about activities, style, etc. that are designated for people based on their biological sex or the gender assigned at birth.

**Genderqueer	A person who does not subscribe to conventional gender norms, identifies as neither male nor female, or a combination of male and female.
*Heteroflexible	One who identifies as predominately heterosexual but may engage in occasional same-sex sexual relations. This is distinct from bisexual where one is attracted to both genders.
*Heteronormative	The assumption that heterosexuality is the normal or preferred sexual orientation, leading to marginalization of any other sexual orientation.
*Internalized Homophobia	Internalizing or taking in society's negative messages about being gay or lesbian. This can lead to self-hatred as well as fear and hatred for gays and lesbians.
***Intersex	An umbrella term for a variety of conditions involving reproductive or sexual anatomy that do not fit the typical (heteronormative) expectations for male or female. May involve hormones, chromosomes, and/or anatomy.
*Lesbian	A woman who is attracted to other women.
**Nonbinary	When a person identifies as something other than their birth gender.
*Pansexual	A person sexually attracted to all/any gender.
*Polyamory	When people have honest, open relationships with more than one partner.
*Sexual Orientation	Describes a person's attraction (physical, sexual, emotional) to others. Sexual orientation includes gay, lesbian, bisexual, pansexual, asexual, and straight/heterosexual. Sexual orientation is often confused with gender identity and they are not the same. For example, one can be a transgender man who is only attracted to other men so would often identify as gay.
**Transgender	A person whose gender identity does not correspond with their biological sex or sex assigned at birth.

* denotes a term related to sexual orientation
** denotes a term related to gender identity
*** neither or both realms

12 Dissociation in Children and Youth

When traumatized children do not learn from past actions and repeatedly engage in destructive behaviors, it is a signal that something is amiss, and it would be wise to explore whether there are dissociated parts that are contributing to, or responsible for, their behavior.

(Frances Waters, 2016)

Dissociation is under-recognized and under-reported in the assessment and treatment of traumatized children and adolescents. The phenomenon of dissociation is complex; thus many definitions of dissociation, and theories about the concept and treatment of dissociation, exist. The complexity may contribute to the lack of awareness and understanding, as well as misdiagnosis and treatment of dissociation in children and adolescents. Although there are similarities to adults in the presentation and symptomology, among youth the developmental processes may lead to different manifestations of dissociation. Also, developmental processes suggest that dissociative youth may be amenable to different treatment interventions than adults. This chapter strives to illuminate the complexity and the importance of recognizing and working with dissociation in youth.

Theories and Definitions of Dissociation

There are numerous theories and models for working with dissociation in adults and youth; however, this chapter focuses primarily on the theory of structural dissociation (van der Hart, Nijenhuis & Steele, 2006). Various definitions of dissociation also exist. We will review some of the definitions and then consider the similarities among definitions. Many experts in the field of trauma and dissociation pay homage to pioneering psychologist Pierre Janet, as he recognized connections between trauma and integrative failure in the early 1900s (e.g. Ogden, Minton & Pain, 2006; van der Hart, Brown & van der Kolk, 1989; Waters, 2016). Van der Kolk & Fisler (1995) described dissociation as "a compartmentalization of experience: elements of the experience are not integrated into a unitary whole, but are stored in memory as isolated fragments consisting of sensory perceptions or affective states" (p. 510). Ogawa et al. (1997) stated that dissociation "refers to a wide variety of behaviors that represent lapses in psychobiological and cognitive processing" (p. 855).

Steele (2013) asserts: "Structural dissociation is a complex developmental deficit in which traumatized children have been unable to adequately integrate their personality and sense of self into a cohesive organization that is stable across time and situations." (p. 5). More recently, Mosquera and Steele (2017) note that literature contains three different categories of experiences referred to as "dissociation": 1) symptoms of absorption and detachment, 2) symptoms of depersonalization and derealization, and 3) division of the personality. Specifically in relation to dissociative youth, Waters (2016) argues that the younger the child, the more prone they are to dissociation because they possess fewer coping skills and there is often no other way to escape the traumatic experience(s); furthermore, dissociation is an instinctive biological response and the most primitive form of self-defense – a freeze mode – when faced with threat or fear of annihilation. According to Spiegel et al. (2011): "Dissociation is a disruption of and/or discontinuity in the normal, subjective integration of one or more aspects of psychological functioning, including—but not limited to—memory, identity, consciousness, perception, and motor control." (p. 826).

Commonalities among definitions are the tendency to split off or compartmentalize components of the traumatic memories, failure to integrate into a cohesive sense of self, dissociation as a disruption of identity/memory/consciousness, fluctuations in mood and behavior, and the primitive nature of dissociation as a defense mechanism. Considering these factors, it is clear that there can be far-reaching consequences of reliance on dissociative tendencies beyond the period of danger and into adulthood.

Wieland (2015) differentiates between three levels of dissociation in children and adolescents: mild, moderate, and severe. In terms of structural dissociation (SD), there are also three levels: primary, secondary, and tertiary. Following are descriptions of the three levels of SD, along with explanations of relevant terms.

Primary SD

With primary SD, there is one ANP (apparently normal personality) that is responsible for going on with daily life activities, and one EP (emotional part of the personality) that contains disowned or split-off emotions or related aspects of a traumatic memory. In my work with dissociative children and youth, I use the acronym WAS (Wise Adolescent Self) instead of ANP. WAS is less pathologizing, and it is easier to say and remember WAS than ANP. The WAS carries on with daily tasks, or inborn action systems (Badenoch, nd; Ogden, 2015; Pietromonaco & Feldman Barrett, 2000; Steele et al., 2010): exploration (school, and possibly work for teens), play, energy regulation (e.g. sleep, eating), social engagement, sexuality and reproduction, attachment, and caregiving. The EPs comprise defense systems: fight, flight, freeze, collapse/feigned death, and attach cry. Each of the EPs has a purpose but all are concerned with protection, boundary-setting and distancing.

In terms of primary SD, then, there may be an EP that holds the freeze response connected to the trauma. The trauma could be a car accident or a single incident of abuse (e.g. hit by a caregiver, attacked at school, date rape). When triggered, the EP (freeze response) may be activated and interfere with the youth's functioning. Fisher (2017) refers to this interference as being hijacked by the EP. Primary SD is also considered a Type I or "small t" trauma. Note that there are two categories of defense response represented in the EPs: mobilizing and immobilizing. Immobilizing defenses typically come into play when a mobilizing defense is not possible (e.g. cannot flee from the attacker) or if fighting back would bring greater harm or compromise attachment to the caregiver (as when the caregiver is also the abuser).

Secondary SD

When there is more trauma, additional EPs may be created. In this case, there is a WAS and several EPs (e.g. fight, flight, and freeze) contain split-off aspects of the trauma. It is easy to see how confusing it would be when there is disruption from various confusing emotions that seem to come out of nowhere, impacting functioning across settings such as school or home. Secondary SD is also referred to as Type II trauma in the literature.

Tertiary SD

Additional WASs may be created when there is prolonged, chronic traumatization. In terms of the DSM-5, this is Dissociative Identify Disorder. This is complex trauma and often involves a relational component. For example, the child may have experienced severe neglect or repeated physical and/or sexual abuse by a caregiver or caregivers. There may be a WAS that deals with home life, and a distinct WAS that goes to school every day. The WASs often have different presentations (e.g. affective, behavioral, cognitive) and may not be aware of each other's existence.

Structural Dissociation in Youth

Childhood and adolescent dissociation is under-recognized and under-reported. While there is an increasing body of literature and research, and dissociation is considered a natural reaction to chronic traumatization in childhood, clinicians may overlook the possibility of dissociation. Fisher (2017) contends that there is a correlation between undiagnosed dissociative disorders and severity of symptoms. A comprehensive trauma assessment that elicits information about possible dissociative processes is an essential first step (European Society on Trauma and Dissociation, 2017; International Society for the Study of Dissociation, 2004; Silberg, 2013; Waters, 2016; Wieland, 2015). If dissociation is overlooked or misdiagnosed, treatment may be ineffective (Waters, 2005a and b).

How Might These Emotional Parts or Defensive Subsystems Manifest in Youth?

Wieland and Silberg (2013) assert: "Dissociation is a psychophysiological process that can protect children facing overwhelming emotions, body sensations, and/or knowledge of those experiences by enabling them to split off and separate these reactions from conscious awareness." The structural dissociation model helps clinicians to conceptualize and work with the "split-off" parts created by the overwhelmed youths' attempt to protect themselves. The visual charts developed by Janina Fisher (2012) reflect secondary SD, and are useful when providing psychoeducation to youth and their caregivers. The SD model itself is useful for psychoeducation and reassuring to clients who worry they are "crazy" (Fisher, 2017). Following is a list of the ways EPs (emotional parts or defensive parts) might show up in youth. Refer to Figure 12.1 for an adaptation of Fisher's (2012) structural dissociation chart for use with youth.

When assessing youth, general warning signs or symptoms of dissociation include the following:

- history of childhood trauma, particularly if relational trauma, or prolonged and chronic trauma;
- history of sexualized, self-harming (e.g. cutting, burning, head-banging, or picking/scratching skin), or violent behavior;
- observe eye movements for fluttering or rolling back in the head;
- blanking out or extended trance states;
- reports of auditory hallucinations, or voices in their head that sound angry or tell them to do things to themselves or others (i.e. persecutory voices);
- memory problems/transient amnesia for huge chunks of time (even years) or events;
- regressed behavior;
- refers to self in the third person (i.e. we);
- imaginary friends/playmates beyond typical age/developmental level (e.g. 10 years of age), and an insistence that they are real;
- depersonalization and/or derealization;
- substance use;
- incongruence of affect or inappropriate response to a situation (e.g. laugh when someone is injured), or rapid and extreme mood changes (e.g. from happy or calm to rage);
- inconsistent performance of abilities across time or situation (e.g. singing, playing a game, piano playing, artistic skills), dramatic changes in preferences (e.g. food, clothing style), or extreme changes in handwriting;
- vehement denials on being accused of lying, even when there are witnesses present, often followed by distress for being accused of something they do not remember doing;
- prone to fantasy and exhibits difficulty connecting to reality (e.g. negatively impacting school or work performance, and this is distressing to the youth).

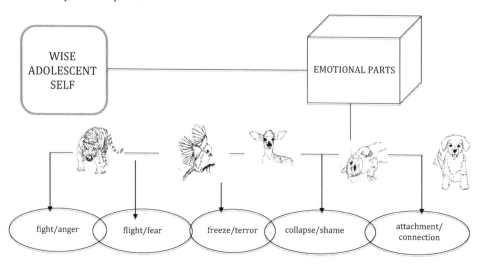

Figure 12.1 Structural Dissociation in Youth
Source: Adapted from Janina Fisher, (2009). *Psychoeducational Aids for Working with Psychological Trauma.* Cambridge, MA: Kendall Press. www.janinafisher.com. Used with permission. Animal art created by Melanie Cheskes MSW, RSW.

Refer to Waters (2016), Silberg (2013), Wieland (2015), ISST-D's Guidelines for the Evaluation and Treatment of Dissociative Symptoms in Children and Adolescents (2004), and ESTD's Guidelines for the Assessment and Treatment of Children and Adolescents with Dissociative Symptoms and Dissociative Disorders (2017) for elaboration of the above warning signs and symptoms.

Treatment of Dissociation in Children and Youth

Phase-oriented treatment, as with complex trauma, is recommended for the treatment of dissociation (Fisher, 2017). Within phase-oriented treatment, or any trauma treatment for that matter, safety and stabilization are paramount (Waters, 2016). If the youth has inadequate coping skills or resources and we begin addressing the trauma, there could be an increase in dissociation or regression to a previous stage of treatment as the youth is overwhelmed by triggers or memories of the trauma.

Treatment Guidelines and Goals

Experts in the field have outlined treatment guidelines, interventions, and goals for working with dissociative youth. Additionally, international associations for the study and treatment of dissociative disorders propose guidelines for working with dissociative youth. You will notice there is overlap and you are invited to consult with each writer's material for elaboration on the points noted.

Table 12.1 The EPs of Structural Dissociation in Children and Youth

SURVIVAL EP	FIGHT	FLIGHT	FREEZE	COLLAPSE/FEIGNED DEATH	ATTACH
PRIMARY EMOTION	*Rage*	*Fear*	*Terror*	*Shame*	*Needy*
MANIFESTATIONS	• Aggression (toward self and others) • Hypervigilance • Critical (of self and others) • Suicidal • Often says No! (tantrums) • Bullies others • Negative self-talk (harsh inner critic) • IBS/disgestive problems	• Alcohol and drug use • Eating disorders • Impulsivity • Risky sex • Inability to commit (e.g. school, relationships) • Inability to trust • Emotional numbing • Runaway • Forgetful/memory problems • Trances or spacing out	• Anxiety or panic attacks • Agoraphobia • Heightened startle response • Selective mutism • Tense body/rigidity	• Depression, hopelessness, despair • Can't say No • "good boy/girl" • Bullied by others • Bowel or bladder incontinence**	• Separation anxiety • Clingy • Regressive • Somatic complaints (e.g. headaches, stomachaches) • Tries to please others

**Bowel and bladder incontinence (known diagnostically as Enuresis and Encopresis) are complicated and likely reflect a plummet from a high arousal freeze defense to a feigned death. However, Encopresis is also about control so may also belong in the Fight column.

In her recently published, comprehensive guide *Healing the Fractured Child: Diagnosis and Treatment of Youth with Dissociation*, Frances Waters (2016) proposes the following overarching treatment principles:

1. Focus on primary trauma-related symptoms rather than secondary symptoms (e.g. behaviors, somatization, low self-esteem).
2. Safety is paramount – this includes physical and psychological safety typically provided in a predictable environment.
3. Recognize that every behavior has purpose or meaning.
4. Educate caregivers and youth about trauma and dissociation.
5. Encourage engagement in developmentally appropriate activities.
6. Engage all parts or aspects of the child in the assessment and treatment process.
7. Encourage responsibility for behaviors across all self-states or parts.
8. Engage caregivers in the assessment and treatment process.
9. Promote attachment between caregiver and the "whole child."
10. Promote metacognition or mentalization – the ability to self-reflect and think about thinking, and to hold conflicting feelings about people or situations.

Joyanna Silberg's work *The Child Survivor: Healing Developmental Trauma and Dissociation* (2013) stipulates the following treatment principles:

1. Maintain an attitude of deep respect for the wisdom of the individual child's coping techniques.
2. Keep a belief in the possibility to heal and the potential for future thriving.
3. Utilize a practical approach to symptom management.
4. Create a relationship of both validation and expectation.
5. Recognize (and help child and caregiver understand) that trauma symptoms are both automatic and learned.
6. The therapeutic relationship – critical in the healing process.

ISST-D (International Society for the Study of Trauma and Dissociation) and ESTD (European Society on Trauma and Dissociation) have similar comprehensive guidelines:

1. Qualifications of Child and Adolescent Practitioners – have an understanding of child development, belong to a regulatory body, participate in ongoing clinical training, remain current with the scientific literature on dissociation, develop collegial relationships and participate in peer supervision or study groups (especially to prevent vicarious traumatization and burnout), and be flexible and creative in using a range of treatment techniques and interventions.
2. Assessment – use screening tests (e.g. A-DES) and diagnostic tests if indicated (e.g. MID), clinical interviews, consider co-morbid conditions, and rule out medical conditions. Ongoing assessment during treatment

is recommended. Note: refer to Chapter 3 (in this book), and the list of warning signs/symptoms above for areas to explore during clinical interviews.

3. Treatment – length and course depends on the individual, the family, and the severity; consider multidisciplinary coordination of care and include collaterals (e.g. teachers, pediatrician) in treatment whenever possible.

4. Role of the therapist – empathic connection with the whole child, demonstrate acceptance of parts of the youth as this facilitates the child's acceptance of disowned parts, balance confidentiality with legal rights of caregivers. Also, recognize role as potentially powerful influence on the youth's behavior – an empathic, nonjudgmental stance may encourage sharing information about the internal factors they understand to be impacting their behaviors and mood. Include family in the treatment whenever possible, and help them understand that the whole child is responsible for behaviors.

5. Encourage child to participate in normalizing activities (e.g. sports, music, or art programs).

6. Therapeutic goals – help child develop sense of cohesiveness (affect, cognitions, behavior), enhance motivation for growth and promote child's belief in own potential, encourage self-acceptance and knowledge about feelings perceived as unacceptable (i.e. disowned or disavowed EPs), help the child resolve conflicting feelings, desensitize trauma memories, correct negative core beliefs about the self (e.g. "I'm bad," I'm unlovable," and feelings of helplessness), help child to monitor and use self-regulation skills, promote healthy attachments and interpersonal connections through effective communication of feelings and needs.

7. Adjunctive treatments – art or music therapy, family therapy, group therapy, pharmacotherapy, educational interventions, inpatient or residential treatment, and referral for individual caregiver treatment if deemed necessary to support child's treatment.

Summary

This chapter contains a lot of information. While there are different theories and guidelines, there are some key points to reflect on. These are the key points that I hope readers take away from this chapter:

1. Conduct a comprehensive trauma assessment, considering past and present factors that may impact the youth's functioning. Think of the four Ps: predisposing, precipitating, perpetuating, and protective. Assessment is an ongoing process to allow monitoring of symptoms and progress.

2. Engage child and caregivers, as well as other significant people or services involved in the child's life, in the assessment and treatment. This helps ensure consistency across settings.

3. Safety and stabilization is paramount and must be considered in all phases of treatment.

4. Psychoeducation is essential for youth and their caregivers. Psychoeducation does the following:
   - validates youth's experience of dissociation as an adaptive coping response to being overwhelmed during the trauma;
   - helps the youth understand the purpose of the disowned emotional parts or defense system;
   - helps the youth and caregiver understand the importance of developing their capacities to co- and self-regulate; and
   - encourages acceptance of the whole child, eliminating the need to fragment parts of the self.

Case illustrations

Dee

As noted previously, Dee had a lot of sadness, confusion, and anger in relation to her family and childhood. She had expressed anger about her mother not protecting her from the early frightening and overwhelming experiences. We worked to prepare Dee to express her feelings and thoughts with her mother, and I met with her mother in advance as well. Dee's mother was fairly dysregulated herself; thus there was a period of meetings to address mother's dysregulation so that she could be fully present for Dee. This was a family with intergenerational trauma and Dee's mother was acknowledged for doing the best she could (note: Dee's mother began seeing her own therapist around this time). Empathy and compassion for mother's experience were critical at this time, not only for mother but also for Dee's healing process. A few months into treatment, Dee was prescribed a mood stabilizer and this seemed to help somewhat with her dysregulation.

When Dee and her mother got together, Dee shrunk into a ball in the corner of the couch and she grabbed a cushion, clutching it close to her body. When they began communicating, Dee's voice was soft and squeaky, and then she broke down into sobs and screamed at her mother for ruining her life. This reaction (e.g. posture, facial expression, tone of voice) had not been observed previously. Dee's mother was attentive, attuned, and unshaken; however, she shared that she had not seen this part of Dee before. At home, mom shared, Dee was aggressive when angry at her (e.g. throwing things, yelling, and swearing), and she was extremely difficult to calm down. Following the rages, Dee retreated into her room and frequently engaged in self-injurious behavior behind closed doors. After her rages, Dee often did not remember the details of the interaction with her mother nor could she recall the details related to cutting herself. Subsequently, we had a few more conjoint sessions and Dee was able to express herself to her mother without cowering, regressing, or sobbing. Between conjoint sessions, psychoeducation about structural dissociation, specifically the EPs (Dee's emerging conflicted fight, collapse, and attach cry), helped Dee experience and accept parts that had split off.

Through talk therapy and somatic interventions, Dee explored the purpose of her emotional parts. She learned that she had cut off feelings of vulnerability and a fight part was used to protect the scared parts of herself. Additionally, Dee learned that a flight part (self-injury and substance use) was typically activated following rage at her caregiver. An understanding of the purpose for the creation of, and hijacking by, the various defense systems allowed Dee to make sense of her experience. Over time, Dee developed skills to tolerate and manage affect that was outside her window of tolerance. She stopped using weed and self-injury to self-soothe, and reported that she was no longer hijacked by the previously disowned emotional parts. Today Dee is functioning well at home and in college, and she is enjoying a healthy intimate relationship.

Lake

Lake was referred to me by a colleague due to the client's complex presentation: issues related to gender identity and dissociation. At our first session, Lake informed me that they were transgender and asked me which pronouns I used. Lake was not receiving any form of hormone (e.g. testosterone) treatment when we met. Also during our first meeting, Lake informed me that they had Dissociative Identity Disorder. Additionally, Lake was identified with learning disabilities, was extremely anxious much of the time, reported self-injurious behavior (cutting and burning, hitting self in the face) and suicidal ideation, and they were being assessed for Autism Spectrum Disorder. In the room, Lake was constantly moving or fidgeting, speech was either tangential and fast-paced or impoverished, and their eye contact alternated between very good to completely absent. Lake's parents were supportive and often accompanied Lake to appointments. Their parents shared that Lake had difficulty with peer relationships at school and they were frequently in trouble at school due to immature, impulsive behavior. At home, their parents noted, Lake kept a trail of knives and other sharp objects between their bed and the bedroom door. Lake expressed disgust about the idea of sex and disliked physical contact of any kind.

As we began to explore some of the school-related problems, Lake expressed having no memory of the immature, impulsive outbursts that led to punishment at school. Nor did they have any recollection of the peer interactions that led to being ostracized by friends. They also had no idea why they felt compelled to place a trail of knives in their bedroom every night before going to sleep. Lake drew the "system" that lived in their head. The system consisted of three floors and 12 distinct parts. Lake used the terms system and parts when they spoke about what was going on inside. The parts varied in age and gender. They were distressed about the voices and the times when parts "fronted," causing them grief in social and school situations. Lake referred to parts taking over as "fronting."

Indeed, Lake presented a complex picture. We completed clinical interviews and screening tests (A-DES); then Lake completed a MASC (Multidimensional Anxiety Scale for Children) and the MID (Multidimensional Inventory of Dissociation). The MID suggested diagnoses of PTSD and DID, along with Borderline Personality traits (severe). There were elevated validity scales on the MID so, as required, we reviewed these areas and items. Lake was aware of their tendency to be attention-seeking and clingy at times. They shared that it seemed impossible for anyone to understand what they felt and experienced inside. Learning about structural dissociation, and dissociation as a result of early childhood trauma, provided a sense of relief and normalization for Lake.

A critical turning point in treatment was Lake's recovered memory of having been sexually assaulted at 5 years of age. Previously, Lake recalled only a fragment of the incident. We spent some time working through this memory, bringing in caregivers for support as needed, and Lake went through a period of grieving the younger girl part's sexual assault. This memory had been fractured off due to intense fear: the older male perpetrator threatened to kill the 5-year-old and tried to drown her in a lake when she screamed. Nobody heard the scream because they were out in a lake at night. The support and validation of Lake's caregiver were important. We were not able to process the memory through somatic means at this time because Lake was still in phase one treatment. At various times in treatment, we checked in with the system. A few weeks after Lake's memory of the near-drowning surfaced, their disowned girl part appeared in the system. We discussed the reappearance of this part of the self and what that meant for Lake. Lake shared that this part felt safe to come out and join the others now.

Lake also had self-destructive (persecutory) and protector parts. Over time (years), using techniques such as Fraser's dissociative table, Lake developed communication and collaboration among parts of their system. We used a team approach (Waters, 2016) as well. We began experimenting with somatic methods to enhance reconnection to the body, increase felt sense of safety (with self and others), and Lake learned and used grounding and containment strategies in various settings. Lake's artistic interests and talents were integrated into treatment frequently as they created concrete reminders of the various strategies. For example, they created painted rocks for grounding (note: different parts had preferences for strategies).

Lake's capacity to self-regulate and integrate parts of themselves were reflected in various areas:

- They stopped laying a knife trail about a year into therapy.
- Lake stopped self-injurious behavior and suicidal ideation ceased.
- Lake no longer has parts "front" and there is rarely any inner chatter.
- Lake's memory problems diminished.
- Lake grew increasingly comfortable with physical contact and began dating a young man.
- Peer relations improved and school-related disruptions disappeared. Lake completed high school and is now attending university.

Appendices

Appendix A: Worksheets

Trauma Assessment – Child/Adolescent

SECTION A

Child's Name	
DOB	
Caregiver/Guardian(s)	
Referral Source	
Child Protection Service Involvement?	
Custody/Adoption?	
Current Living Situation/Family Constellation	
Cultural/Religious	
School/Grade	
IEP/Special Ed?	
Other Providers?	

Child's Perception of Presenting Situation
Caregiver Perception

SECTION B

Previous Services/Service Providers			
Date(s)	Agency/Person	Type of Service	Details

Other Current Providers (e.g. Pediatrician, Psychiatrist)

Current/Past Medication(s)?
Current
Previous

Allergy Information

Medical/Surgical/Hospitalization History

Developmental History	
Pregnancy/Birth	
Milestones	
Language	
Cognitive	
Academic	
Motor/Coordination	
Social	
Other	

SECTION C

Family History – complete and attach genogram	
Caregiver/Guardian Relationship History	
Communication Style	
Discipline Style	
Moves (freq./reason)	
Extended Family Relationships	
Sibling Relationships	
Substance Abuse	
Mental Illness	
Medical Conditions	
Legal Involvement	
Other	

SECTION D

Abuse/Trauma History – circle and provide details	
None physical neglect verbal emotional domestic violence exposure sexual abuse	
Victim of	
Victim of	
Engaged in Acts of	
Significant Separation/Loss	

Substance Use/Addictions – list substance, age of first and last use, frequency, any adverse effects (include cigarettes, alcohol, weed, internet, gambling, sex, etc.)	

SECTION E

MSE
Interaction
friendly   cooperative   hostile/angry   anxious   evasive   detached   guarded   bored other_____
Motor activity
Normal   hyperactive   listless   fidgety   slowed   facial tics   body tics   other_____
Affect
Full range/approp to content incongruent flat labile intense/reactive
Other_____
Perceptual disturbance
No evidence of psychosis hallucinations (audio/visual) delusional/magical thinking other_____
Orientation
Person   place   time   situation
Appearance
Neat/clean unkempt   heavy thin   average weight   poor hygiene other
Speech

SECTION F

	Areas of Concern – circle past or present and provide details		
past present	Aggression/violence toward others	past present	Self-injury
past present	Property destruction	past present	Suicidal thoughts/talk/attempts
past present	Anxious/panic attacks	past present	Eating disorder/binging/purging/picky
past present	Sleep disturbance/nightmares	past present	Depressed mood/sadness
past present	Hallucinations/delusions/paranoia	past present	Fire-setting or cruelty to animals
past present	Social withdrawal/isolation	past present	Rapid mood changes
past present	Homicidal thoughts/behavior	past present	Sexual concerns
past present	Truancy/academic concerns	past present	Impulsive/inattentive/distractible
past present	Running away	past present	Legal issues
past present	Stealing/vandalism	past present	Obsessive/compulsive behavior
past present	Needs to be in control	past present	Enuresis/Encopresis
past present	Body image	past present	Aversion to touch/sensory issues
past present	Self-concept	past present	Other

SECTION G

	Skills/Abilities – check and provide details as relevant		
	Personal hygiene		Family resources
	Household chores		Coping skills/emotional management
	Nutrition		Leisure/recreation
	Personal safety		
	Other		

Resources – check and provide details as relevant		
	Housing		Healthcare
	Transportation		Family/social
	Educational		Community involvement/support
	Financial		Other

Regulation	
	Able to tolerate and express strong emotions such as anger, frustration, sadness. Please provide details.
	Able to tolerate and manage conflict. Please provide details.
	Able to self-soothe. Please provide details.
	Able to form and maintain healthy relationships, and demonstrates awareness of age-appropriate boundaries. Please provide details.

SECTION H

Strengths
Individual/family strengths (per child):
Individual/family strengths (per caregiver):
Protective factors:
Interests:
Three wishes:

My Sensory Record

Building Block	Touch	Taste	Sound	Smell	Sight
5-sense Perception					
Sensation(s) & Location(s)					
Feeling(s)					
Thought(s)					

Client:

	Date/Details	Date/Details	Date/Details
Defense/Boundaries			
Containment			
Alignment			
Centering			
Locomotion/Movement			
Interactive Regulation			
Grounding			
Posture			
Breath			
Developmental Movements			

Appendix B: Resources for Working with Traumatized Youth and Their Caregivers

Breathwork Books (Young Children)

1. *Six Healing Sounds: Qigong for Children* – Lisa Spillane (2011)
2. *Breathe! Tai Chi Qigong for Children* – Linda Tenenbaum (2012)
3. *Boy and a Bear* – Lori Lite (1996)
4. *Peaceful Piggy Meditation* – Kerry Lee MacLean (2006)

Mindfulness Books (Range of Ages)

1. *Puppy Mind* – Andrew Jordan Nance (2016)
2. *Sitting Still Like a Frog: Mindfulness Exercises for Kids (and Their Parents)* – Eline Snel (2013)
3. *Self-Compassion and Mindfulness for Teens Card Deck: 54 Exercises and Conversation Starters* – Lee-Anne Gray (2017)
4. *Still Quiet Place: A Mindfulness Program for Teaching Children and Adolescents to Ease Stress and Difficult Emotions* – Amy Saltzman (2014)
5. *Mindful Movements: Ten Exercises for Well-Being* – Thich Nhat Hahn (2008)
6. *Dialectical Behavior Therapy Skills. 101 Mindfulness Exercises and Other Fun Activities for Children and Adolescents: A Learning Supplement* – Gage Riddoch, Julie Eggers Huber, and Kimberly Christensen (2009)

Books on Feelings and/or Sensations

1. Anne Westcott's series of books – trained in SP and EMDR among other methods to treat young traumatized children. Books include *How Little Coyote Found His Secret Strength: A Story About How to Get Through Hard Times* (2017), and *Bomji and Spotty's Frightening Adventure: A Story About How to Recover from a Scary Experience* (2017)
2. *Listening to My Body: A Guide to Helping Kids Understand the Connection Between Their Sensations (What the Heck Are Those?) and Feelings So That They Can Get Better at Figuring out What They Need* – Gabi Garcia (2017)

3. Jan Yordy has developed books, games, and DVDs to help children and caregivers understand feelings and sensations, and she offers a variety of therapeutic tools (such as EFT, Brain Gym) to facilitate growth, https://energyconnectiontherapies.com/educational-resources/

Psychoeducational Material about Brain Development and Trauma

1. Janina Fisher's Psychoeducational Flipchart – https://janinafisher.com/flip-chart
2. *Brain Puzzle and Model – W. W. Norton* (2008)
3. *Human Anatomy Brain Model – Learning Resources*

Games

1. Yoga Pretzels – Tara Guber (2005)
2. The Kids' Yoga Deck – Annie Buckley (2003)
3. Yoga Poses for Kids, Deck One – Gisele Shardlow (2015), (https://shop.kidsyogastories.com/products/yoga-poses-for-kids-cards-deck-one)
4. Too Close, Too Far, Just Right: A Game About Personal Space (used for working with physical boundaries) – Sandra Singer, Lois Feigenbaum, and Claudia Weiss (n.d.)
5. Mindful Games Activity Cards: 55 Fun Ways to Share Mindfulness with Kids and Teens (2017)
6. Talking, Feeling and Doing Game – Richard Gardner (n.d.)

Audio, Video and Social Media, and Resourceful Websites

1. LifeMath – interactive kids' computer-based programs
2. *Still Quiet Place: Mindfulness for Teens* by Amy Saltzman
3. *Still Quiet Place: Mindfulness for Young Children* by Amy Saltzman
4. Bellaruth Naparstek's website Health Journeys (e.g. www.healthjourneys.com/audio-library/teen-stress-anxiety-depression/meditations-for-teens)
5. Yoga Poses for Kids, www.namastekid.com/tools/type/kids-yoga-poses/
6. Lee Holden's qigong videos, www.holdenqigong.com/
7. Jacob Hamm – excellent animations on attunement, attachment, and trauma (YouTube), great for clinicians and psychoeducation for youth and caregivers
8. Post-traumatic Growth Inventory, www.emdrhap.org/content/wp-content/uploads/2014/07/VIII-B_Post-Traumatic-Growth-Inventory.pdf
9. The Professional Quality of Life measure (ProQOL) is owned by the Center for Victims of Torture (www.CVT.org) and distributed free of charge for noncommercial usage. The ProQOL is updated periodically and multiple translations are available. Please check www.ProQOL.org for the most recent version and to request permission to use the ProQOL for research purposes.
10. Biodots: biofeedback skin thermometers, https://biodots.net/

Appendix C: Flashback and Nightmare Protocols, Self-Regulation Checklist for Caregivers

Flashback Protocol

Right now I am feeling _____,
                 name a feeling, like scared

and sense _____, _____ in my
        name 2 things happening inside your body, like shaking or hot/cold

body because I am remembering _____.
           name the event with using a word or 2

I am looking around where I am now in _____ in
               this year

_____,
     the place you are now

and I can see _____, _____, _____
         name 3 things you see right now in this room or place

So I know _____ is not happening anymore and I am safe.
    name the event again, using a word or two.

Adapted from Rothschild, B. (2000). *The Body Remembers: The Psychophysiology of Trauma and Trauma Treatment*. New York: W. W. Norton, p. 133.

Nightmare Protocol

If I wake up after a nightmare feeling _____,

name a feeling, like scared

and notice _____ in my body

name what is happening inside, like shaking or hot/cold

because I just had a bad dream about _____,

name the nightmare using a word or

two

I will look around where I am now in _____ in my

this year

_____.

room, like bedroom or living room.

As I look around and see _____, I

name 3 things you see right now in this room

will know I am awake and safe and the nightmare is not happening anymore.

Adapted from Rothschild, B. (2000). *The Body Remembers: The Psychophysiology of Trauma and Trauma Treatment*. New York: W. W. Norton, p. 134.

How Do You Self-Regulate?

Created by Angie Voss, OTR, ASensoryLife.com (used with permission, all rights reserved)

Understanding how you as an adult self-regulate will help you to better understand and support your child's sensory needs for self-regulation. These are just some common strategies we use as humans...the possibilities are endless! There is no right or wrong answer and this is not a test or assessment; it is a self-awareness tool. The more items you check in a certain section will help you determine which sensory systems you use most often to self-regulate.

This list may be reprinted for educational purposes with reference and credit to the author and website listed above. Thank you!

Do you use movement to self-regulate? (vestibular input)

Check all that apply

- Get up and down often while working or shift position and squirm around a lot
- Tilt back on 2 legs of the chair
- Prefer a swivel and leaning back type chair or ball chair
- Enjoy running, jogging, biking, and other movement based sports
- Roll neck and head around all of the time
- Prefer to stand to work or read something
- Prefer rocking chairs and gliders
- Love to swing any chance you get
- Always moving, prefer to move vs. sit
- Very fidgety while seated
- Pace back and forth

Do you use proprioception and/or deep pressure touch to self-regulate?

Check all that apply

- Enjoy housework and vacuuming
- Enjoy gardening
- Enjoy yoga
- Tap toe, heel, foot
- Like lifting weights and other hard work activities
- Cross your legs when seated
- Tap your pen or pencil
- Often twisting, stretching your body
- Love cozy heavy blankets
- Love massages
- Enjoy hanging on bars or tree limbs any chance you get
- Enjoy wrestling and rough housing

- Love tight and cozy spaces
- Love to cuddle
- Love big squeezes and hugs
- Cracks knuckles and joints
- Clenching jaw
- Need heavy blankets or being tightly tucked in to sleep well
- Love to be wrapped in blankets
- Take deep breaths often

Do you use tactile input to self-regulate?

Check all that apply

- Love having your back rubbed with light touch
- Enjoy it when someone plays with your hair
- Twist and twirl your own hair
- Scratch, rub, and pick at your own skin
- Pick your nose (yuck, I know!)
- Love to pet animals
- Always exploring textures of clothing, fabric on furniture, or pillows
- Click pens, play with paper clips
- Always like something in your hand to fidget with such as knitting or other craft

Do you use auditory input to self-regulate?

Check all that apply

- Enjoy listening to music
- Whistle or hum while you work
- Prefers a quiet and calm space to attend to a task
- Needs background noise to work
- Tap objects or fingers, hands, toes to a certain beat
- Likes white noise

Do you use visual input to self-regulate?

Check all that apply

- Enjoy watching water features and fountains
- Find fish tanks soothing
- Love lava lamps and other visually stimulating toys and objects
- Prefer a very tidy space in order to work
- Very organized, dislike clutter
- Find certain colors very soothing and calming
- Prefer things to match just right in color

- Like to line things up (or even tidy up the shelves at the grocery store!)
- Something out of place or out of sort bothers you
- Do you find this purple form soothing and comforting?
- Do you find this purple form overwhelming and irritating?

Do you use oral sensory and gustatory input to self-regulate?

Check all that apply

- Bite fingernails
- Love to chew gum
- Make clicking sounds or other mouth sounds
- Chew on own hair or pen or something else while working
- Love crunchy or chewy snacks
- Crave salty or spicy foods
- Enjoy drinking through a straw or other resistive type straw such as a CamelBak water bottle
- Bite inside of cheeks or chew on tongue
- Always moving your jaw around
- Smoke cigarettes
- Clear throat often
- Lick lips often
- Emotional eating

Do you use olfactory input (smell) to self-regulate?

Check all that apply

- Enjoy essential oils
- Love scented candles
- Love perfume
- Smell clothing and other fabric type objects
- Enjoy air fresheners
- Love scented markers and erasers
- Love smelling flowers and things in nature
- Love smelling different foods

References

Abendroth, M. & Figley, C. (2013). Vicarious Trauma and the Therapeutic Relationship. Retrieved from www.researchgate.net/profile/CR_Figley/publication/259609739_Vicarious_Trauma_and_the_Therapeutic_Relationship/links/5550b09f08ae956a5d25d123/Vicarious-Trauma-and-the-Therapeutic-Relationship.pdf.

Abram, K.M., Teplin, L.A., Charles, D.R., Longworth, S., McClelland, G. & Dulcan, M. (2004). Posttraumatic Stress Disorder and Trauma in Youth in Juvenile Detention. *Archives of General Psychiatry.* 61:4.

Afifi, T., MacMillan, H., Boyle, M., Taillieu, T., Cheung, K. & Sareen, J. (2014). Child Abuse and Mental Disorders in Canada. *Canadian Medical Association Journal.* 186:9.

Ainsworth, M., Blehar, M., Waters, E. & Wall, S. (1978). *Patterns of Attachment: A Psychological Study of the Strange Situation.* Hillsdale, NJ: Erlbaum.

American Academy of Child and Adolescent Psychiatry (2012). A Guide for Community Child-Serving Agencies on Psychotropic Medications for Children and Adolescents. Retrieved from www.aacap.org/App_Themes/AACAP/docs/press/guide_for_community_child_serving_agencies_on_psychotropic_medications_for_children_and_adolescents_2012.pdf.

American Psychiatric Association. (2013). *Diagnostic and Statistical Manual of Mental Disorders, Fifth Edition.* Washington, DC: American Psychiatric Association.

Anda, R., Felitti, V., Bremner, D., Walker, J, Whitfield, C., Perry, B., Dube, S. & Giles, W. (2006). The Enduring Effects of Abuse and Related Adverse Experiences in Childhood: A Convergence of Evidence from Neurobiology and Epidemiology. *European Archives of Psychiatry and Clinical Neuroscience.* 256:3.

Andersen, J. & Blosnich, J. (2013). Disparities in Adverse Childhood Experiences among Sexual Minority and Heterosexual Adults: Results from Multi-State Probability-Based Sample. *PLoS One.* 8:1.

Andersen, J., Zou, C. & Blosnich, J. (2015). Multiple Early Victimization Experiences as a Pathway to Explain Physical Health among Sexual Minority and Heterosexual Individuals. *Social Science & Medicine.* 133.

Aposhyan, S. (2004). *Body Mind Psychotherapy.* New York: W. W. Norton.

Arvidson, J., Kinniburgh, K., Howard, K., Spinazzola, J., Strothers, H., Evans, M., Andres, B., Cohen, C. & Blaustein, M. (2011). Treatment of Complex Trauma in Young Children: Developmental and Cultural Considerations in Application of the ARC Intervention Model. *Journal of Child and Adolescent Trauma,* 4:1.

Austin, A., Herrick, H. & Proescholdbell, S. (2015). Adverse Childhood Experiences Related to Poor Adult Health among Lesbian, Gay, and Bisexual Individuals. *AJPH Research*. 106:2.

Badenoch, B. (n.d.). *How Understanding Our Embodied Brains Can Support Lives of Hope and Resilience*. Louisville, CO: Sounds True.

Badenoch, B. (2008). *Being a Brain-Wise Therapist: A Practical Guide to Interpersonal Neurobiology*. New York: W. W. Norton.

Badenoch, B. (2018). *The Heart of Trauma: Healing the Embodied Brain in the Context of Relationships*. New York: W. W. Norton.

Bainbridge Cohen, B. (2012). *Sensing, Feeling and Action*. Northampton, MA: Contact Editions.

BC Provincial Mental Health and Substance Use Planning Council. (2013). Trauma-Informed Practice Guide. Retrieved from www.bccewh.bc.ca.

Becerra-Culqui, T., Liu, Y., Nash, R., Cromwell, L, Flanders, W., Getahun, D., Giammettei, S., Hunkeler, E., Lash, T., Millman, A., Quinn, V., Robinson, B., Roblin, D., Sandberg, D., Silverberg, M., Tangpricha, V. & Goodman, M. (2018). Mental Health of Transgender and Gender Nonconforming Youth Compared with Their Peers. *Pediatrics*. 141:5.

Beetz, A., Uvnäs-Moberg, K., Julius, H. & Kotrschal, K. (2012). Psychosocial and Psychophysiological Effects of Human-Animal Interactions: The Possible Role of Oxytocin. *Frontiers in Psychology*. 3:234.

Blaustein, M. & Kinneburgh, K. (2010). *Treating Traumatic Stress in Children and Adolescents: How to Foster Resilience Through Attachment, Self-Regulation and Competence*. New York: Guilford.

Bombay, A., Matheson, K. & Anisman, H. (2013). The Intergenerational Effects of Indian Residential Schools: Implications for the Concept of Historical Trauma. *Transcultural Psychiatry*. 51:3.

Bontempo, D. & D'Augelli, A. (2002). Effects of At-School Victimization and Sexual Orientation on Lesbian, Gay or Bisexual Youths' Health Risk Behavior. *Journal of Adolescent Health*. 30:5.

Boon, S., Steele, K. & van der Hart, O. (2011). *Coping with Trauma-Related Dissociation: Skills Training for Patients and Therapists*. New York: W. W. Norton.

Bowlby, J. (1973). *Attachment and Loss: Volume 2*. New York: Basic Books.

Briggs, P., Hayes, S. & Changaris, M. (2018). Somatic Experiencing® Informed Therapeutic Group for the Care and Treatment of Biopsychosocial Effects upon a Gender Diverse Identity. *Frontiers in Psychiatry*. 9:53.

Bromberg, P. (2006). *Awakening the Dreamer: Clinical Journeys*. Mahwah, NJ: Analytic Press.

Bryn Austin, S., Ziyadeh, N., Corliss, H., Rosario, M., Wypij, D., Haines, J., Camargo, C. & Field, A. (2009). Sexual Orientation Disparities in Purging and Binge Eating from Early to Late Adolescence. *Journal of Adolescent Health*. 45:3.

Cary, C. & McMillen, C. (2012). The Data behind the Dissemination: A Systemic Review of Trauma-Focused Cognitive Behavioral Therapy for Use with Children and Youth. *Children and Youth Services Review*. 34:4.

Causadias, J., Salvatore, J. & Sroufe, A. (2012). Early Patterns of Self-Regulation and Risk and Promotive Factors in Development: A Longitudinal Study from Childhood to Adulthood in a High-Risk Sample. *International Journal of Behavioral Development*. 36:4.

Clark, B. (2017). Ethics in Youth Care Practice with Transgender Youth. *International Journal of Child, Youth and Family Studies*. 8:1.

Clark, C., Classen, C., Fourt, A. & Shetty, M. (2015). *Treating the Trauma Survivor: An Essential Guide to Trauma-Informed Care*. New York: Routledge/Taylor & Francis Group.

Classen, C., Gronskaya Palesh, O. & Aggarwal, R. (2005). Sexual Revictimization: A Review of the Empirical Literature. *Trauma, Violence, & Abuse*. 6:2.

Clements-Nolle, K., Lensch, T., Baxa, A., Gay, C., Larson, S. & Yang, W. (2018). Sexual Identity, Adverse Childhood Experiences, and Suicidal Behaviors. *Journal of Adolescent Health*. 62.

Cloitre, M. (2015). The "One Size Fits All" Approach to Trauma Treatment: Should We Be Satisfied? *European Journal of Psychotraumatology*. 6.

Cloitre, M., Stolbach, B., Herman, J., van der Kolk, B., Pynoos, R., Wang, J. & Petkova, E. (2009). A Developmental Approach to Complex PTSD: Childhood and Adult Cumulative Trauma as Predictors of Complexity. *Journal of Traumatic Stress*. 22:5.

Cohen, J., Mannarino, A. & Deblinger, E. (2006). *Treating Trauma and Traumatic Grief in Children and Adolescents*. New York: Guilford.

Cohen, J., Mannarino, A., Kliethermes, M. & Murray, L. (2012). Trauma-Focused CBT for Youth with Complex Trauma. *Child Abuse and Neglect*. 36:6.

Columbia University's Mailman School of Public Health (2007). Gay Men Have Higher Prevalence of Eating Disorders. *Science Daily*. April 14. Retrieved January 9, 2019 from www.sciencedaily.com/releases/2007/04/070413160923.htm.

Cook, A., Spinazzola, J., Ford, J., Lanktree, C., Blaustein, M., Cloitre, M., DeRosa, R., Hubbard, R., Kagan, R., Liautaud, J., Mallah, K., Olafson, E. & van der Kolk, B. (2005). Complex Trauma in Children and Adolescents. *Psychiatric Annals*. 35:390–398.

Courtois, C. (2004). Complex Trauma, Complex Reactions: Assessment and Treatment. *Psychotherapy: Theory, Research, Practice, Training*. 41:4.

Courtois, C.A. & Ford, J.D. (eds.). (2009). *Treating Complex Traumatic Stress Disorders: An Evidence-Based Guide*. New York: Guilford.

Cozolino, L. (2006). *The Neuroscience of Human Relationships: Attachment and the Developing Social Brain*. New York: W. W. Norton.

De Bellis, M. & Zisk, A. (2014). The Biological Effects of Childhood Trauma. *Child and Adolescent Psychiatric Clinics of North America*. 23:2.

Dennison, P. & Dennison, G. (1992). *Brain Gym: Simple Activities for Whole Brain Learning*. Ventura, CA: Edu-Kinesthetics, Inc.

De Young, A., Kenardy, J. & Cobham, V. (2011). Trauma in Early Childhood: A Neglected Population. *Clinical Child and Family Psychological Review*. 14:231–250.

Diemer, E., Grant, J., Munn-Chernoff, M., Patterson, D. & Duncan, A. (2015). Gender Identity, Sexual Orientation, and Eating-Related Pathology in a National Sample of College Students. *Journal of Adolescent Health*. 57.

Dieterich-Hartwell, R. (2017). Dance/Movement Therapy in the Treatment of Post Traumatic Stress: A Reference Model. *The Arts in Psychotherapy*. 54.

Doctor, Fariya. (2018). Interview, June 28.

Doidge, N. (2007). *The Brain That Changes Itself*. New York: Penguin.

Doidge, N. (2015). *The Brain's Way of Healing: Remarkable Discoveries and Recoveries from the Frontiers of Neuroplasticity*. New York: Penguin.

Dolan, Y. (1991). *Resolving Sexual Abuse*. New York: W. W. Norton.

Dreikurs, R. (1991). *Children: The Challenge. The Classic Work on Improving Parent–Child Relations*. New York: Plume Books.

Emerson, D. (2015). *Trauma-Sensitive Yoga in Therapy: Bringing the Body into Treatment*. New York: W. W. Norton.

European Society on Trauma and Dissociation. (Updated July 2017). *Guidelines for the Assessment and Treatment of Children and Adolescents with Dissociative Symptoms and Dissociative Disorders*. Retrieved from www.estd.org/sites/default/files/files/estd_guidelines_child_and_adolescents_first_update_july_2.pdf.

Everall, R. & Paulson, B. (2004). Burnout and Secondary Traumatic Stress: Impact on Ethical Behaviour. *Canadian Journal of Counselling*. 38:1.

Fay, D. (2017). *Attachment-Based Yoga and Meditation for Trauma Recovery*. New York: W. W. Norton.

Feldenkrais, M. (1990). *Awareness Through Movement*. New York: HarperCollins.

Felitti, V. & Anda, R. (2005). *The ACE Study*. DVD series produced by Cavalcade Productions.

Felitti, V., Anda, R., Nordenberg, D., Williamson, D., Spitz, A., Edwards, V., Koss, M. & Marks, J. (1998). Relationship of Childhood Abuse and Household Dysfunction to Many of the Leading Causes of Death in Adults: The Adverse Childhood Experiences (ACE) Study. *American Journal of Preventive Medicine*. 14:4.

Figley, C. (2002). Compassion Fatigue: Psychotherapists' Chronic Lack of Self-Care. *JCLP: In Session: Psychotherapy in Practice*. 58:11.

Figley, C. & Figley, K. (2017). *Compassion Fatigue Resilience*. In Seppala, E.M., Simon-Thomas, E., Brown, S.L., Worline, M.C. Cameron, C.D. & Doty, J.R. (eds.). *The Oxford Handbook of Compassion Science*. Downloaded July 2018 from Oxford Handbooks Online, www.oxfordhandbooks.com.

Fisher, J. (n.d.). The Treatment of Structural Dissociation in Chronically Traumatized Patients. Retrieved from https://janinafisher.com/resources.

Fisher, J. (1999). The Work of Stabilization in Trauma Treatment. Paper presented at the Trauma Center Lecture Series 1999. Retrieved February 2018 from https://janinafisher.com.

Fisher, J. (2000). Adapting EMDR Techniques in the Treatment of Dysregulated or Dissociative Patients. Paper presented at the International Society for the Study of Dissociation Annual Meeting, San Antonio, TX.

Fisher, J. (2010). Brain to Brain: The Therapist as Neurobiological Regulator. *Psychotherapy Networker*. 34:1.

Fisher, J. (2012). *Psychoeducational Aids for Working with Psychological Trauma*. Watertown, MA: Center for Integrative Healing.

Fisher, J. (2017). *Healing the Fragmented Selves of Trauma Survivors: Overcoming Internal Self-Alienation*. New York: Routledge.

Fisher, J. (2017). Trauma-Informed Stabilisation Treatment: A New Approach to Treating Unsafe Behaviour. *Australian Clinical Psychologist*. 3:1. Retrieved from https://janinafisher.com/pdfs/2017-tist-australian-psychologist.pdf.

Ford, J.D. & Courtois, C.A. (eds.). (2013). *Treating Complex Traumatic Stress Disorders in Children and Adolescents: Scientific Foundations and Therapeutic Models*. New York: Guilford.

Ford, J., Grasso, D., Greene, C., Levine, J., Spinazzola, J. & van der Kolk, B. (2013). Clinical Significance of a Proposed Developmental Trauma Disorder Diagnosis: Results of an International Survey of Clinicians. *Journal of Clinical Psychiatry*. 74:8.

Geller, S. & Porges, S. (2014). Therapeutic Presence: Neurophysiological Mechanisms Mediating Feeling Safe in Therapeutic Relationships. *Journal of Psychothearpy Integration*. 24:3.

Gendlin, E. (1978). *Focusing*. New York: Bantam-Dell.

Gene-Cos, N., Fisher, J., Ogden, P. & Cantrel, A. (2016). Sensorimotor Psychotherapy Group Therapy in the Treatment of Complex PTSD. *Annals of Psychiatry and Mental Health.* 4:6.

Goddard-Blyth, S. (2011). *Genius of Natural Childhood: The Secrets of Thriving Children.* Gloucestershire, UK: Hawthorne.

Goldstein, B. & Siegel, D. (2013). The Mindful Group: Using Mind–Body–Brain Interactions in Group Therapy to Foster Resilience and Integration. In Siegel, D. & Solomon, M. (eds.), *Healing Moments in Psychotherapy.* New York: W. W. Norton.

Government of Canada (2013). Aboriginal Children: The Healing Power of Cultural Identity. Retrieved from www.canada.ca/en/public-health/services/health-promotion/childhood-adolescence/programs-initiatives/aboriginal-head-start-urban-northern-communities-ahsunc/aboriginal-children-healing-power-cultural-identity.html.

Grant, J., Mottet, L., Tanis, J., Herman, J., Harrison, J. & Keisling, J. (2010). National Transgender Discrimination Survey Report on Health and Heath Care. Retrieved from www.thetaskforce.org/static_html/downloads/resources_and_tools/ntds_report_on_health.pdf.

Grant, J., Mottet, L., Tanis, J., Harrison, J., Herman, J. & Keisling, J. (2011) Injustice at Every Turn: A Report of the National Transgender Equality and National Gay and Lesbian Task Force. Retrieved from www.thetaskforce.org/static_html/downloads/reports/reports/ntds_full.pdf.

Gray, P. (2011). The Decline of Play and the Rise of Psychopathology in Children and Adolescents. *American Journal of Play.* 3:4.

Hart, H. & Rubia, K. (2012) Neuroimaging of Child Abuse: A Critical Review. *Frontiers in Human Neuroscience.* 6:52, 1–24.

Haskell, L. (2003). *First Stage Trauma Treatment: A Guide for Mental Health Professionals Working with Women.* Toronto, ON: Centre for Addiction and Mental Health.

Heitzler, M. (2013). Broken Boundaries, Invaded Territories: The Challenges of Containment in Trauma Work. *International Body Psychotherapy Journal.* 12:1.

Heller, L. & LaPierre, A. (2012). *Healing Developmental Trauma: How Early Trauma Affects Self-Regulation, Self-Image, and the Capacity for Relationship.* Berkeley, CA: North Atlantic Books.

Herman, J. (1992). Complex PTSD: A Syndrome in Survivors of Prolonged and Repeated Trauma. *Journal of Traumatic Stress.* 5:3.

Herman, J. (1992). *Trauma and Recovery.* New York: Basic Books.

Hodgdon, H., Blaustein, M., Kinniburgh, K., Peterson, M. & Spinazzola, J. (2015) Application of the ARC Model with Adopted Children: Supporting Resiliency and Family Well-Being. *Journal of Child and Adolescent Trauma.* 9:1.

Hottes, T., Bogaert, L., Rhodes, A., Brennan, D. & Gesink, D. (2016). Lifetime Prevalence of Suicide Attempts among Sexual Minority Adults: A Systematic Review and Meta-analysis. *AJPH Research.* 106:5.

House, A., Van Horn, E., Coppeans, C. & Stepleman, L. (2011). Interpersonal Trauma and Discriminatory Events as Predictors of Suicidal and Nonsuicidal Self-Injury in Gay, Lesbian, Bisexual, and Transgender Persons. *Traumatology.* 17:2.

Hyatt-Burkhart, D. (2014). The Experience of Vicarious Posttraumatic Growth in Mental Health Workers. *Journal of Loss and Trauma: International Perspectives on Stress & Coping.* 19:5.

Iacoboni, M. (2008). *Mirroring People: The Science of Empathy and How We Connect with Others.* New York: Picador.

Iacoboni, M. & Mazziotta, J. (2007). Mirror Neuron System: Basic Findings and Clinical Applications. *Annals of Neurology.* 62:3.

International Society for the Study of Dissociation. (2004). Guidelines for the Evaluation and Treatment of Dissociative Symptoms in Children and Adolescents. *Journal of Trauma & Dissociation.* 5:3.

Irwin, J. & Austin, E. (2013). Suicide Ideation and Suicide among White Southern Lesbians. *Journal of Gay and Lesbian Mental Health.* 17:4.

James, B. (1989). *Treating Traumatized Children.* New York: The Free Press.

Janet, P. (1925). *Psychological Healing: A Historical and Clinical Study.* Translated from the French by Eden and Cedar Paul. London: George Allen & Unwin, Ltd. New York: Macmillan Company. Retrieved from www.archive.org.

Jensen, T., Holt, T., Ormhaug, S., Egeland, K., Granly, L., Hoaas, L. & Wentzel-Larsen, T. (2014). A Randomized Effectiveness Study Comparing Trauma-Focused Cognitive Behavioral Therapy with Therapy as Usual for Youth. *Journal of Clinical Child & Adolescent Psychology.* 43:3.

Jirek, S. (2015). Soul Pain: The Hidden Toll of Working with Survivors of Physical and Sexual Violence. Retrieved from www.researchgate.net/publication/282070580_Soul_Pain_The_Hidden_Toll_of_Working_With_Survivors_of_Physical_and_Sexual_Violence.

Johanson, G. (2009). Psychotherapy, Science and Spirit: Nonlinear Systems, Hakomi Therapy, and the Tao. *Journal of Spirituality in Mental Health.* 11:3.

Kagan, R., Lautaud, J., Mallah, K., Olafson, E. & van der Kolk, B. (2005). Complex Trauma in Children and Adolescents. *Psychiatric Annals.* 35:5.

Kaiser, E., Gillette, C. & Spinazzola, J. (2010). A Controlled Pilot-Outcome Study of Sensory Integration (SI) in the Treatment of Complex Adaptation to Traumatic Stress. *Journal of Aggression, Maltreatment & Trauma.* 19.

Keating, L. & Muller, R. (2018) *LGBTQ+ People's Experiences of Accessing Trauma Therapy.* Paper presented at the International Society for Trauma and Dissociation. Chicago, IL.

Kellerman, N. (2013). Epigenetic Transmission of Holocaust Trauma: Can Nightmares Be Inherited? *Israel Journal of Psychiatry and Related Sciences.* 50.

Konanur, S., Muller, R., Cinamon, J., Thornback, K. & Zorzella, K. (2015). Effectiveness of Trauma-Focused Cognitive Behavioral Therapy in a Community-Based Program. *Child Abuse & Neglect.* 50:157–170.

Kozlowska, K., Walker, P., McLean, L. & Carrive, P. (2015). Fear and the Defense Cascade: Clinical Implications and Management. *Harvard Review of Psychiatry.* 23:4.

Krasner, M., Epstein, R., Beckman, H., Suchman, A., Chapman, B., Mooney, C. & Quill, T. (2009). Association of an Educational Program in Mindful Communication with Burnout, Empathy, and Attitudes among Primary Care Physicians. *Journal of the American Medical Association.* 302:12.

Kugler, B., Bloom, M., Kaercher, L, Truax, T. & Storch, E. (2012). Somatic Symptoms in Traumatized Children and Adolescents. *Clinical Psychiatry and Human Development.* 43:.

Langmuir, J., Kirsh, S. & Classen, C. (2012). A Pilot Study of Body-Oriented Group Psychotherapy: Adapting Sensorimotor Psychotherapy for the Group Treatment of Trauma. *Psychological Trauma: Theory, Research, Practice, and Policy.* 4:2.

Lanius, R., Vermetten, E. & Pain, C. (eds.). (2010). *The Impact of Early Trauma on Health and Disease.* Cambridge, UK: Cambridge University Press.

LeDoux, J. (1996). *The Emotional Brain: The Mysterious Underpinnings of Emotional Life.* New York: Touchstone.

Lee M.S., Pittler, M.H. & Ernst, E. (2007). External Qigong for Pain Conditions: A Systematic Review of Randomized Clinical Trials. *Journal of Pain*. 8.

Levine, P. (2008). *Healing Trauma: A Pioneering Program for Restoring the Wisdom of Your Body*. Boulder, CO: Sounds True.

Levine, P. (2013). *Creating Safety in Practice: How the Right Tools Can Speed Healing and Reduce Symptoms for Even the Most Traumatized Clients*. NICABM Webinar.

Levine, P. (2015). *Memory and Trauma: Brain and Body in a Search for the Living Past*. Berkeley, CA: North Atlantic Books.

Malchiodi, C. & Crenshaw, D. (eds.). (2014). *Creative Arts and Play Therapy for Attachment Problems*. New York: Guilford.

Mannarino, A., Cohen, J., Deblinger, E., Runyon, M. & Steer, R. (2012). Trauma-Focused Cognitive-Behavioral Therapy for Children: Sustained Impact of Treatment 6 and 12 Months Later. *Child Maltreatment*. 17:3.

Mark-Goldstein, B. & Ogden, P. (2013). Sensorimotor Psychotherapy as a Foundation of Group Therapy with Younger Clients. In *The Interpersonal Neurobiology of Group Psychotherapy and Group Process*. New York: Routledge.

Marks, R. (2017). Qigong Exercise and Arthritis. *Medicines*. 4:4.

Mate, G. (2003). *When the Body Says No: The Cost of Hidden Stress*. Toronto, ON: Random House.

Mathieu, F. (2012). *The Compassion Fatigue Workbook: Creative Tools for Transforming Compassion Fatigue and Vicarious Traumatization*. New York: Routledge/Taylor and Francis Group.

May-Benson, T. (2016). A Sensory Integration-Based Intervention to Trauma-Informed Care for Children. *OTA The Koomar Center White Paper*. Newton, MA: OTA The Koomar Center.

Middleton, J. & Potter, C. (2015). The Relationship between Vicarious Trauma and Turnover among Child Welfare Professionals. *Journal of Public Child Welfare*. 9.

Mosquera, D. & Steele, K. (2017). Complex Trauma, Dissociation and Borderline Personality Disorder: Working with Integrative Failures. *European Journal of Trauma & Dissociation*. 1:63–71.

Muller, R., Vascotto, N.A., Konanaur, S. & Rosenkranz, S. (2013). Emotion Regulation and Psychopathology in a Sample of Maltreated Children. *Journal of Child & Adolescent Trauma*. 6:1, 25–40.

Musicaro, R., Spinazzola, J., Arvidson, J., Swaroop, S., Goldblatt Grace, L., Yarrow, A., Suvak, M. & Ford, J. (2017). The Complexity of Adaptation to Childhood Polyvictimization in Youth and Young Adults: Recommendations for Multidisciplinary Responders. *Trauma, Violence & Abuse*. 20:1.

Mustanski, B., Garofalo, R. & Emerson, E. (2010). Mental Health Disorders, Psychological Distress, and Suicidality in a Diverse Sample of Lesbian, Gay, Bisexual, and Transgender Youths. *American Journal of Public Health*. 100:12.

Nadal, K., Issa, M., Leon, J., Meterko, V., Widerman, M. & Wong, Y. (2011). Sexual Orientation Microaggressions: "Death by a Thousand Cuts" for Lesbian, Gay, and Bisexual Youth. *Journal of LGBT Youth*. 8:3.

National Child Traumatic Stress Network. (2012). ARC: Attachment, Self-Regulation, and Competency Fact Sheet. Retrieved from www.nctsn.org/sites/default/files/interventions/arc_fact_sheet.pdf.

National Child Traumatic Stress Network. (2014). *LGBTQ Youth and Sexual Abuse: Information for Mental Health Professionals*.

Newcomb, M., Heinz, A. & Mustanski, B. (2012). Examining Risk and Protective Factors for Alcohol Use in Lesbian, Gay, Bisexual, and Transgender Youth: A Longitudinal Multilevel Analysis. *Journal of Studies on Alcohol and Drugs.* 73.

Nijenhuis, E. & van der Hart, O. (2011). Dissociation in Trauma: A New Definition and Comparison with Previous Formulations. *Journal of Trauma and Dissociation.* 12:416–445.

Nijenhuis, E., van der Hart, O. & Steele, K. (2010). Trauma-Related Structural Dissociation of the Personality. *Activitas Nervosa Superior.* 52:1.

Odendaal, J. & Meintjes, R. (2003). Neurophysiological Correlates of Affiliative Behaviour between Humans and Dogs. *Veterinary Journal.* 165.

Ogawa, J., Sroufe, A., Weinfield, N., Carlson, E. & Egeland, B. (1997). Development of the Fragmented Self: Longitudinal Study of Dissociative Symptomology in a Nonclinical Sample. *Development and Psychopathology.* 9:.

Ogden, P. (2009). Modulation, Mindfulness and Movement in the Treatment of Trauma-Related Depression. In Kerman, M. (ed.), *Clinical Pearls of Wisdom.* New York: W. W. Norton.

Ogden, P. (2012) *Level 1: Training in Affect Dysregulation, Survival Defenses, and Traumatic Memory.* Broomfield, CO: Sensorimotor Psychotherapy Institute.

Ogden, P. (2014). In White, K. (ed.), Wisdom of the Body, Lost and Found. London: Karnac Books.

Ogden, P. (2015). Proximity, Defence and Boundaries with Children and Care-Givers: A Sensorimotor Psychotherapy Perspective. *Children Australia.* 40.

Ogden, P. & Fisher, J. (2007). The Movements of Play: Restoring Spontaneity and Flexibility in Traumatized Individuals. *GAINS Quarterly.*

Ogden, P. & Fisher, J. (2015). *Sensorimotor Psychotherapy: Interventions for Trauma and Attachment.* New York: W. W. Norton.

Ogden, P., Goldstein, B. & Fisher, J. (2012). Brain-to-Brain, Body-to-Body: A Sensorimotor Perspective on the Treatment of Children and Adolescents. In Longo, R. E. et al. (eds.), *Current Perspectives and Applications in Neurobiology: Working with Young People Who Are Victims and Perpetrators of Sexual Violence.* Holyoke, MA: Negri Press. Retrieved from www.drbonniegoldstein.com/wp-content/uploads/2016/01/Ogden-Goldstein-Fisher-Brain-to-Brain-Body-to-Body-A-Sensorimotor-Psychotherapy-Perspective-on-the-Treatment-of-Children-and-Adolescents.pdf.

Ogden, P. & Minton, K. (2000). Sensorimotor Psychotherapy: One Method for Processing Traumatic Memory. *Traumatology.* 6:3. Article 3.

Ogden, P., Minton, K. & Pain, C. (2006). *Trauma and the Body: A Sensorimotor Approach to Psychotherapy.* New York: W. W. Norton.

Ogden, P., Pain, C., Minton, K. & Fisher, J (2005). The Body in Mainstream Psychotherapy for Traumatized Individuals. *American Psychological Association.* Retrieved from www.sensorimotorpsychotherapy.org/article%20APA.html.

Osofsky, J. (2011). *Clinical Work with Young Traumatized Children.* New York: Guilford.

Panksepp, J. (2003). "Laughing Rats" and the Evolutionary Antecedents of Human Joy? *Physiology and Behavior.* 79.

Panksepp, J. (2010). Science of the Brain as a Gateway to Understanding Play: An Interview with Jaak Panksepp. *American Journal of Play.* Winter.

Pereira, H. (2016). Internalized Homophobia and Suicidal Ideation among LGB Youth. *African Journal of Psychiatry.* 18:2.

Pereira, H. & Rodrigues, P. (2015). Internalized Homophobia and Suicidal Ideation among LGB Youth. *African Journal of Psychiatry.* 18:2.

Perrin, E. (2002). *Sexual Orientation in Child and Adolescent Health Care*. New York: Kluwer Academic Press.

Perry, B. (2006). Applying Principles of Neurodevelopment to Clinical Work with Maltreated and Traumatized Children: The Neurosequential Model of Therapeutics. In Boyd Webb, N. (ed.), *Working with Traumatized Youth in Child Welfare*. New York: Guilford.

Perry, B. (2008). Child Maltreatment: A Neurodevelopmental Perspective on the Role of Trauma and Neglect in Psychopathology. In Beauchaine, T.P. & Hinshaw, S.P. (eds.), *Child and Adolescent Psychopathology*. Hoboken, NJ: Wiley & Sons.

Perry, B. (2009). Examining Child Maltreatment Through a Neurodevelopmental Lens: Clinical Applications of the Neurosequential Model of Therapeutics. *Journal of Trauma and Loss*. 14.

Perry, B. (2014). The Cost of Caring: Secondary Traumatic Stress and the Impact of Working with High-Risk Children and Families. Child Trauma Academy. Retrieved from https://childtrauma.org/wp-content/uploads/2014/01/Cost_of_Caring_Secondary_Traumatic_Stress_Perry_s.pdf.

Perry, B. & Hambrick, E. (2006). The Neurosequential Model of Therapeutics. Retrieved from www.researchgate.net/publication/237346956_The_Neurosequential_Model_of_Therapeutics.

Perry, B. & Pollard, D. (1997). Altered Brain Development Following Global Neglect in Early Childhood. Society for Neuroscience: Proceedings from Annual Meeting, New Orleans. Retrieved from https://childtrauma.org/.

Perry, B. & Szalavitz, M. (2006). *The Boy Who Was Raised as a Dog*. New York: Basic Books.

Perry, B. & Szalavitz, M. (2011). *Born for Love: Why Empathy Is Essential – and Endangered*. New York: William Morrow.

Perry, B., Pollard, R., Blakely, T., Baker, W. & Vigilante, D. (1995). Childhood Trauma, the Neurobiology of Adaptation, and "Use-dependent" Development of the Brain: How "States" Become "Traits." *Infant Mental Health Journal*. 16:4.

Pietromonaco, P. & Feldman Barrett, L. (2000). The Internal Working Models Concept. *Review of General Psychology*. 4:2.

Porges, S. (2011). *The Polyvagal Theory: Neurophysiological Foundations of Emotions Attachment Communication*. New York: W. W. Norton.

Porges, S. (2011). Somatic Perspectives in Psychotherapy. Transcript from Somatic Perspectives Series. www.SomaticPerspectives.com.

Porges, S. (2017). *The Pocket Guide to Polyvagal Theory*. New York: W. W. Norton.

Ramirez de Arellano, M., Lyman, D., Jobe-Shields, L., George, P., Dougherty, R., Daniels, A., Sushmita, S., Huang, L. & Delphin-Rittmon, M. (2014). Trauma-Focused Cognitive-Behavioural Therapy for Children and Adolescents: Assessing the Evidence. *Psychiatric Services*. 65:5.

Rivera, M. (2002). Informed and Supportive Treatment for Lesbian, Gay, Bisexual and Transgendered Trauma Survivors. *Journal of Trauma and Dissociation*. 3:4. (Copy of article provided by Dr. Rivera.)

Roberts, A., Bryn Austin, S., Corliss, H., Vandermorris, A. & Koenen, K. (2010). Pervasive Trauma Exposure among US Sexual Orientation Minority Adults and Risk of Posttraumatic Stress Disorder. *American Journal of Public Health*. 100:12.

Roberts, A., Rosario, M., Corliss, H., Koenen, K. & Bryn Austin, S. (2012). Childhood Gender Nonconformity: A Risk Indicator for Childhood Abuse and Posttraumatic Stress in Youth. *Pediatrics*. 129:3.

Roberts, A., Rosario, M., Slopen, N., Calzo, J. & Bryn Austin, S. (2013). Childhood Gender Nonconformity, Bullying Victimization, and Depressive Symptoms Across Adolescents and Early Adulthood: An 11-Year Longitudinal Study. *Journal of American Child and Adolescent Psychiatry*. 52:2.

Roberts, N. (2009). Early Intervention Following Traumatic Events. *Psychiatry*. 8:8.

Rosenberg, S. (2017). *Accessing the Healing Power of the Vagus Nerve*. Berkeley, CA: North Atlantic Books.

Rothschild, B. (2000). *The Body Remembers: The Psychophysiology of Trauma and Trauma Treatment*. New York: W. W. Norton.

Rothschild, B. (2017). *The Body Remembers, Vol. 2: Revolutionizing Trauma Treatment*. New York: W. W. Norton.

Rubens, L., Felix, E. & Hambrick, E. (2018). A Meta-analysis of the Impact of Natural Disasters on Internalizing and Externalizing Behavior Problems in Youth. *Journal of Traumatic Stress*. 31:3.

Ryan, C., Russell, S., Huebner, D., Diaz, R. & Sanchez, J. (2010). Family Acceptance in Adolescence and the Health of LGBT Young Adults. *Journal of Child and Adolescent Psychiatric Nursing*. 23:4.

Salston, M. & Figley, C. (2003). Secondary Traumatic Stress Effects of Working with Survivors of Criminal Victimization. *Journal of Traumatic Stress*. 16:2.

Saxe, G., Ellis, B.H. & Kaplow, J. (2007). *Collaborative Treatment of Traumatized Children and Teens*. New York: Guilford.

Scaer, R. (2007). *The Body Bears the Burden: Trauma, Dissociation and Disease*. New York: Howarth Medical Press.

Schacter, Miriam. (July 2018). Personal communication.

Schore, A. (1999). *Affect Regulation and the Origin of the Self: The Neurobiology of Emotional Development*. Hillsdale, NJ: Lawrence Erlbaum Associates, Inc..

Schore, A. (2000). Attachment and the Regulation of the Right Brain. *Attachment & Human Development*. 2:1.

Schore, A. (2001). Effects of a Secure Attachment Relationship on Right Brain Development, Affect Regulation and Infant Mental Health. *Infant Mental Health Journal*. 22:1–2.

Schore, A. (2009). Right Brain Affect Regulation. Retrieved from www.allanschore.com/pdf/__SchoreFosha09.pdf.

Shirk, S., Karver, M. & Brown, R. (2011). The Alliance in Child and Adolescent Psychotherapy. *Psychotherapy*. 48:1.

Siegel, D.J. (1999). *The Developing Mind*. New York: Guilford.

Siegel, D. (2007). *The Mindful Brain: Reflection and Attunement in the Cultivation of Well-Being*. New York: Norton.

Siegel, D. (2010). *The Mindful Therapist*. New York: W. W. Norton/Mind Your Brain, Inc.

Siegel, D. (2012). *Pocket Guide to Interpersonal Neurobiology*. New York: W. W. Norton/Mind Your Brain, Inc.

Siegel, D. & Hartzell, M. (2003). *Parenting from the Inside Out*. New York: Penguin.

Siegel, D. & Solomon, M. (eds.). (2013). *Healing Moments in Psychotherapy*. New York: W. W. Norton.

Silberg, J. (2013). *The Child Survivor: Healing Developmental Trauma and Dissociation*. New York: Routledge.

Silkenbeumer, J., Schiller, E., Holdynski, M. & Kartner, J. (2016). The Role of Co-Regulation for the Development of Social-Emotional Competence. *Journal of Self-Regulation and Regulation*. 2.

Smith, S. (2007). Making Sense of Multiple Informants in Child and Adolescent Psychopathology. *Journal of Psychoeducational Assessment*. 25:2.

Snell, R. (2017). Therapist Qualities, Interventions, and Perceived Outcomes: Bringing Developmental Movement into Body Psychotherapy. *International Body Psychotherapy Journal*. 16 supplement.

Spengler, E., Miller, D. & Spengler, P. (2016). Microaggressions: Clinical Errors with Sexual Minority Clients. *Psychotherapy*. 55:3.

Spiegel, D., Loewenstein, R., Lewis-Fernandez, R., Sar, V., Simeon, D., Vermetten, E., Cardena, E. & Dell, P. (2011). Dissociative Disoders in DSM-5. *Depression and Anxiety*. 28.

Spinazzola, J. (2016). JRI presentation, July 29, 2016. Retrieved from YouTube.

Spinazzola, J., Rhodes, A., Emerson, D., Earle, E. & Monroe, K. (2011). Application of Yoga in Residential Treatment of Traumatized Youth. *Journal of the American Psychiatric Nurses Association*. 17:6.

Spinazzola, J., Hodgdon, H., Liang, L., Ford, J., Layne, C., Pynoos, R., Briggs, E. & Stolbach, B. (2014). Unseen Wounds: The Contribution of Psychological Maltreatment to Child and Adolescent Mental Health and Risk Outcomes. *Psychological Trauma: Theory, Research, Practice, and Policy*. 6:S1.

Sprang, G., Clark, J. & Whitt-Woosley, A. (2007). Compassion Fatigue, Compassion Satisfaction, and Burnout: Factors Impacting a Professional's Quality of Life. *Journal of Loss and Trauma*. 12.

Sroufe, L.A. (1995). *Emotional Development: The Organization of Emotional Life in the Early Years*. Cambridge, UK: Cambridge University Press.

Sroufe, L.A. (2005). Attachment and Development: A Prospective, Longitudinal Study from Birth to Adulthood. *Attachment & Human Development*. 7:4.

Stats Canada (2016). Cyberbullying and Cyberstalking among Internet Users Aged 15 to 29 in Canada. Retrieved July 2018 from www150.statcan.gc.ca/n1/en/catalogue/75-006-X201600114693.

Steele, K. (2013). Six Reasons to Assess and Treat Dissociation. *Paradigm*. 18.

Steele, K, van der Hart, O. & Nijenhuis, E. (2005). Phase-Oriented Treatment of Structural Dissociation in Complex Traumatization: Overcoming Trauma-Related Phobias. *Journal of Trauma and Dissociation*. 6:3.

Steele, K., van der Hart, O. & Nijenhuis, E. (2010). Trauma-Related Structural Dissociation of the Personality. *Activitas Nervosa Superior*. 52:1.

Stein, P. & Kendall, J. (2003). *Psychological Trauma and the Developing Brain: Neurologically Based Interventions for Troubled Children*. New York: Routledge.

Steiner-Adair, C. & Barker, T. (2013). *The Big Disconnect: Protecting Childhood and Family Relationships in the Digital Age*. New York: Harper.

Taliaferro, L. & Muehlenkamp, J. (2016). Nonsuicidal Self-Injury and Suicidality among Sexual Minority Youth: Risk Factors and Protective Connectedness Factors. *American Pediatrics*. 17:7.

Tedeschi, R.G. & Calhoun, L.G. (1996). The Posttraumatic Growth Inventory: Measuring the Positive Legacy of Trauma. *Journal of Trauma Stress*. 9:3.

Teicher, M., Anderson, S., Polcari, A., Anderson, C., Navalta, C. & Kim, D. (2003). The Neurobiological Consequences of Early Stress and Childhood Maltreatment. *Neuroscience and Biobehavioral Reviews*. 27:1–2.

The Professional Quality of Life measure (ProQOL) is owned by the Center for Victims of Torture (www.CVT.org) and distributed free of charge for non-commercial usage. The ProQOL is updated periodically and multiple translations are available. Please check www.ProQOL.org for the most recent version and to request permission to use the ProQOL for research purposes.

Trevarthen, C., Delafield-Butt, J.T. & Schögler, B. (2011). Psychobiology of Musical Gesture: Innate Rhythm, Harmony and Melody in Movements of Narration. In Gritten, A. & King, E. (eds.), *Music and Gesture II*. Aldershot: Ashgate.

Tyler, K. & Schmitz, R. (2018). A Comparison of Various Forms of Trauma in the Lives of Lesbian, Gay, Bisexual and Heterosexual Homeless Youth. *Journal of Trauma and Dissociation*. 19:4.

Van der Hart, O., Brown, P. & van der Kolk, B. (1989). Pierre Janet's Treatment of Post-traumatic Stress. *Journal of Traumatic Stress*. 2:4.

Van der Hart, O., Nijenhuis, E. & Steele, K. (2005). Dissociation: An Insufficiently Recognized Major Feature of Complex PTSD. *Journal of Traumatic Stress*. 18:5.

Van der Hart, O., Nijenhuis, E. & Steele, K. (2006). *The Haunted Self: Structural Dissociation and the Treatment of Chronic Traumatization*. New York: W. W. Norton.

Van der Hart, O., Nijenhuis, E., Steele, K. & Brown, D. (2004). Trauma-Related Dissociation: Conceptual Clarity Lost and Found. *Australian and New Zealand Journal of Psychiatry*. 38.

van der Kolk, B. (1989). The Compulsion to Repeat the Trauma. *Psychiatric Clinics of North America*. 12:2.

van der Kolk, B. (1994). The Body Keeps the Score: Memory and the Evolving Psychobiology of Post Traumatic Stress. *Harvard Review of Psychiatry*. 1:5.

van der Kolk, B. (2003). The Neurobiology of Childhood Trauma and Abuse. *Child and Adolescent Psychiatric Clinics of North America*. 12:2.

van der Kolk, B. (2014). *The Body Keeps the Score: Brain, Mind and Body in the Healing of Trauma*. New York: Viking.

van der Kolk, B. & Fisler, R. (1995). Dissociation and the Fragmentary Nature of Traumatic Memories: Overview and Exploratory Study. *Journal of Traumatic Stress*. 8:4.

van der Kolk, B., McFarlane, A. & Weisaeth, L. (eds.). (1996). *Traumatic Stress: The Effects of Overwhelming Experience on Mind, Body, and Society*. New York: Guilford.

van der Kolk, B., Stone, L., West, J., Rhodes, A., Emerson, D., Suvak, M. & Spinazzola, J. (2014). Yoga as an Adjunctive Treatment for Posttraumatic Stress Disorder: A Randomized Controlled Trial. *Journal of Clinical Psychiatry*. 75:6.

Van Dernoot Lipsky, L. (2009). *Trauma Stewardship: An Everyday Guide to Caring for Self While Caring for Others*. San Francisco, CA: Barrett-Koehler Publishers, Inc.

Walters, K.L., Mohammed, S.A., Evans-Campbell, T., Beltra'n, R.E., Chae, D.H. & Duran, B. (2011). Bodies Don't Just Tell Stories, They Tell Histories. *Du Bois Review: Social Science Research on Race*. 8:1. Retrieved from https://pdfs.semanticscholar.org.

Warner, E., Spinazzola, J. & Price, M. (2017). The Boy Who Was Hit in the Face: Somatic Regulation and the Processing of Preverbal Complex Trauma. *Journal of Adolescent Trauma*. 10.

Warner, E., Cook, A., Westcott, A. & Koomar, J. (2012). *SMART: Sensory Motor Arousal Regulation Treatment Manual*. Brookline, MA: The Trauma Center at JRI.

Warner, E., Koomar, J., Lary, B. & Cook, A. (2013). Can the Body Change the Score? Application of Modulation Principles in the Treatment of Traumatized Adolescents in Residential Settings. *Journal of Family Violence.* 28:7.

Warner, E., Spinazzola, J., Westcott, A., Gunn, C. & Hodgdon, H. (2014) The Body Can Change the Score: Empirical Support for Somatic Regulation in the Treatment of Traumatized Adolescents. *Journal of Child and Adolescent Trauma.* 9:4.

Waters, F. (2005a). Recognizing Dissociation in Preschool Children. *ISSD News.* 23:4.

Waters, F. (2005b). When Treatment Fails with Traumatized Children…Why? *Journal of Trauma and Dissociation.* 6:1.

Waters, F. (2016). *Healing the Fractured Child: Diagnosis and Treatment of Youth with Dissociation.* New York: Springer.

Wieland, S. (1997). *Hearing the Internal Trauma: Working with Children and Adolescents Who Have Been Sexually Abused.* Thousand Oaks, CA: Sage.

Wieland, S. (1998). *Techniques and Issues in Abuse-Focused Therapy with Children and Adolescents.* Thousand Oaks, CA: Sage.

Wieland, S. (ed.). (2015). *Dissociation in Traumatized Children and Adolescents,* 2nd edition. New York: Routledge.

Wieland, S. (2017). *Parents Are Our Other Client: Ideas for Therapists, Social Workers, Support Workers, and Teachers.* New York: Routledge.

Yack, Ellen. (2016). Personal communication, April 27.

Yap, A., Ang, S. & Kwan, Y. (2017). A Systematic Review of the Effects of Active Participation in Rhythm-Centred Music Making on Different Aspects of Health. *European Journal of Integrative Medicine.* 9.

Yehuda, R. & Bierer, L. (2009). The Relevance of Epigenetics to PTSD: Implications for the DSM-V. Journal of Traumatic Stress. 22:5. Retrieved from www.ncbi.nlm.nih.gov/.

Zou, C. & Andersen, J. (2015). Comparing the Rates of Early Childhood Victimization Across Sexual Orientations: Heterosexual, Lesbian, Gay, Bisexual, and Mostly Heterosexual. *PLoS One.* 10:10.

Index

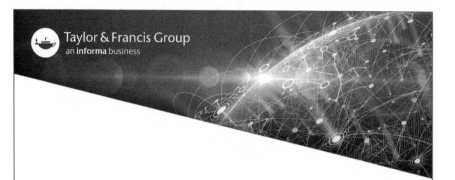